BLESSED DAYS OF ANAESTHESIA

BLESSED DAYS OF ANAESTHESIA

. . . .

How Anaesthetics Changed the World

STEPHANIE J. SNOW

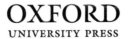

OXFORD
UNIVERSITY PRESS

OXFORD
UNIVERSITY PRESS

Great Clarendon Street, Oxford OX2 6DP

Oxford University Press is a department of the University of Oxford.
It furthers the University's objective of excellence in research, scholarship,
and education by publishing worldwide in

Oxford New York

Auckland Cape Town Dar es Salaam Hong Kong Karachi
Kuala Lumpur Madrid Melbourne Mexico City Nairobi
New Delhi Shanghai Taipei Toronto

With offices in

Argentina Austria Brazil Chile Czech Republic France Greece
Guatemala Hungary Italy Japan Poland Portugal Singapore
South Korea Switzerland Thailand Turkey Ukraine Vietnam

Oxford is a registered trade mark of Oxford University Press
in the UK and in certain other countries

Published in the United States
by Oxford University Press Inc., New York

© Stephanie Snow, 2008

British Library Cataloguing in Publication Data
Data available

Library of Congress Cataloging in Publication Data
Data available

Printed in Great Britain
on acid-free paper
by Clays Ltd, St Ives plc

ISBN 978-0-19-280586-7

1 3 5 7 9 10 8 6 4 2

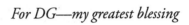

For DG—my greatest blessing

ACKNOWLEDGEMENTS

This book is a further fruit of a project generously supported by a Research Fellowship from the Wellcome Trust for the History of Medicine, undertaken at the Centre for the History of Science, Technology, and Medicine at the University of Manchester. Many institutions have provided invaluable help over the years and I particularly thank staff of the Wellcome Institute for the History of Medicine, the Royal College of Surgeons of England, the British Medical Association, the Royal Society of Medicine, St George's Hospital, St Bartholomew's Hospital, King's College Hospital, the London Hospital, the Royal Free Hospital, the London Metropolitan Archives, Westminster Medical Society, Edinburgh Public Record Office, Glaxo Wellcome, the History of Anaesthesia Society, the John Rylands University Library, and the Liverpool Medical Institute. Sources that I particularly drew on in the preparation of this book are mentioned in Further Reading but I am in debt to many more historians of medicine and other scholars whose work and ideas have sustained my own. I am particularly grateful to Lucy Bending for discussions on ideas of pain in the nineteenth century; Peter Drury for advice on aspects of twentieth-century anaesthesia; Charles Suckling for sharing his memories of the discovery of halothane; and David Watts for giving permission to reprint his poem 'Starting the IV: Anesthesia'. My thanks to those who have read parts, or all of this book, and whose thoughts and helpful criticisms have improved its clarity and accuracy: Emm Barnes, Peter Drury, John Pickstone, Charles Suckling, and Meriel Underwood. Special thanks go to Emm Barnes for timely and sustaining support. I am grateful to my editors at Oxford University Press: Marsha Filion, whose enthusiasm for the project started the ball rolling; and Latha Menon and James Thompson, whose well-judged nudges kept it going. Finally, but most importantly, I thank my family, especially Evie, Verity, and Gwyn, who have tolerated the writing process with cheerful forbearance.

Stephanie J. Snow
Erway Hall
December 2007

CONTENTS

LIST OF ILLUSTRATIONS

PREFACE

Pain is a universal experience. Few readers of these pages can have escaped the discomfort of headaches, toothaches, or indeed the debilitating pain of chronic conditions such as arthritis or backache. In the Western world we have easy access to a wide range of analgesics and anaesthetics. Some conditions remain impervious to treatment but most sufferers will find relief of some sort. Certainly no patient will have to undergo a surgical operation without anaesthesia, nor women face childbirth without the option of pain relief. Medical schools teach students that alleviating physical pain is central to all specialties and there is an enormous amount of evidence-based literature which shows the benefits of different therapies.

Our understandings of pain are very different to those which dominated medicine before the introduction of anaesthesia in the 1840s. Then, although practitioners had always sought to alleviate suffering, pain was widely thought to be of physiological and moral value. In surgery, pain was the stimulant that preserved life in the body during the stress of an operation. Understandings of pain had begun to change in the eighteenth century, but the pain of operations seemed intransigent until the discovery of anaesthesia. We might imagine that soon after William Morton demonstrated the anaesthetic properties of ether in Massachusetts General Hospital in October 1846, every patient subsequently undergoing an operation received pain relief. But this was not so: the introduction of anaesthesia was controversial. In Britain, from December 1846 until at least the 1860s, anaesthesia was a selective practice: many patients continued to endure pain and suffering during operations.

Anaesthesia challenged Victorian understandings of pain at the most fundamental level. What was its purpose? How could medical control of suffering be reconciled with the Christian view that human pain was God's will? Doctors, clergymen, and writers debated the subject passionately. Because inhaling ether and chloroform could be fatal, it struck deep into one of medicine's central questions: what were the risks versus benefits of medical intervention? By the end of the nineteenth century anaesthesia was a routine part of surgery. What had seemed radical in the 1840s—suspending the pain of an operation—had become commonplace.

This book is the story of how that happened. It tells of the discoveries of the anaesthetic properties of ether, chloroform, and nitrous oxide, and the debates about its risks in surgery, in childbirth, and on the battlefield. It also reveals chloroform's dark associations with crime and, indeed, murder. Many of its characters could appear on a soap opera cast list: American dentists Horace Wells, Charles Jackson, and William Morton, pivotal figures in the discovery of nitrous oxide's and ether's anaesthetic properties in the 1840s who became embroiled in a bitter and long-lasting feud over priority; John Snow, a Yorkshire lad made good as a London general practitioner, architect of the scientific principles of anaesthesia, and champion of anaesthetic inhalers; James Young Simpson, one of Edinburgh's most popular physicians, discoverer of the anaesthetic properties of chloroform in November 1847, and supporter of a 'simple hanky' for administering chloroform. And of course Queen Victoria, who contributed to the saga when she used chloroform during the birth of Prince Leopold in April 1853. These human dramas mark the highs and lows of one of medicine's most important discoveries.

But at a deeper level, it is a story of changing Western attitudes to pain which had far-reaching social and cultural consequences. Anaesthesia showed how pain could be suspended during operations without adversely affecting the patient's well being; it gradually eroded the argument that pain was necessary and functional in surgery. In this way it enabled the profound change in medical and social attitudes to pain which had begun in the eighteenth century to be realized. The new view that physical suffering could and should be prevented where possible spread outwards from surgery to medicine where it intensified the attention given to the palliation of pain in chronic disease and death. Beyond medicine, anaesthesia became a touchstone for humanitarianism, fuelling public distaste of pain and concern about the morality of inflicting suffering. It is no coincidence that from the 1860s onwards public executions became private events, legislation was introduced to reduce cruelty to animals in scientific experiments, and ideas of pain in Christian doctrine were reworked.

As the century drew to a close, the jubilees of the discovery of ether and chloroform were celebrated in 1896 and 1897. Doctors agreed that anaesthesia was one of the century's most important discoveries. The surgeon, wrote *The Times* in 1897, is no longer a butcher but an artist: 'a skilled user of the finest tools' who with the benefit of anaesthesia could practise 'the scientific conservation of life and structure and function'. Science, as we shall see through the story of John Snow, had played its part in establishing anaesthesia. But what patients found most irresistible was the humane way in which anaesthesia relieved pain and suffering. This book's title originates from Charles Darwin's reference to 'the blessed days of chloroform'. It could equally well have been chosen from other patient accolades: 'the greatest blessing of this age', Fanny Longfellow; 'miraculous and merciful', Charles Dickens, 'delightful beyond measure', Queen Victoria. Despite the risk of death from anaesthesia, thousands of patients breathed ether, chloroform, and nitrous oxide, believing themselves to be living in a world better than the one into which they had been born. Later generations, including ourselves, took for granted that surgery would be pain free and that doctors would use their skills and resources to palliate pain.

The establishment of anaesthesia recast understandings of pain irrevocably. It is almost impossible for us to imagine a time when painful operations were the norm, and hardly surprising that anaesthesia was ranked in the top three of medical breakthroughs since 1840, in a 2007 poll organized by the *British Medical Journal*. It is a story which affects each of us. Few readers would quibble with Darwin's words; many will have had experience of anaesthesia, or know someone who has. To see how much anaesthesia changed the world, we need to understand a little about matters in the eighteenth century, the time when understandings of pain began to shift.

1

· · · ·

INTRODUCTION

Fanny Burney was no stranger to pain. Best known for her novel *Evelina,* published in 1778, Fanny suffered from mastitis after the birth of her son, Alex, in December 1794. The pain was so intense 'as to make life—even my happy life—scarce my wish to preserve!' she wrote. Little did she know then that seventeen years later she would have to bear a mastectomy without pain relief. Her description of the operation, undertaken in Paris, is a moving testimony to the awful suffering patients endured in operations without anaesthesia. The first indication of the problem was a 'small pain' in her breast. Reluctant to seek medical advice, she was eventually persuaded by her husband, M. d'Arblay, to consult M. Dubois, the surgeon who had treated her for the breast abscess. Dubois' opinion was that 'a small operation would be necessary to avert evil consequences.' 'My dread & repugnance, from a thousand reasons *besides* the pain, almost shook all my faculties, &, for some time, I was rather confounded & stupefied than affrighted,' Fanny recalled. As 'the pains became quicker & more violent' she sought a second opinion. M. Larrey, recently awarded a baronetcy for his services to Napoleon's armed forces, prescribed a new regime of therapies which brought some improvement. However, his concern was strong enough to ask for a further opinion from the anatomist Dr Ribe and, as a last resort, Dr Moreau, a physician. But to no avail. After a final consultation between the doctors, Fanny was summoned to attend them. Seeing Larrey shrinking behind the sofa she realized 'all hope was over ... I now saw it was inevitable, and abstained from any further effort. ... I was formally condemned to an operation.' The doctors were unequivocal about the severity of the forthcoming operation: 'vous souffrirez *beaucoup*', warned Dubois. Ribe charged Fanny to cry and scream during surgery; any attempt to restrain herself could have serious consequences, he warned. But Dubois and Larrey refused to give Fanny more than four hours notice of the operation. They wanted to limit her anxiety, they said. When operations were performed at home, patients' families often attended, but M. d'Arblay was too agitated; the doctors refused to have him present. To keep Fanny's fears in check, a closet in the house was secretly filled with dressings, bandages, and compresses. Fanny made her will and appointed two women to attend her during the procedure. On the morning of 30 September 1811 Fanny received a letter from Larrey giving her two hours notice of the operation. 'I will not be ready until 1 o'clock,' she protested; in the event Dubois was delayed until 3 o'clock. Fanny waited; 'the sight of the immense quantity of bandages, compresses, sponges, Lint —made me a little sick,' she wrote. Finally '7 Men in black' entered the salon. Dubois took charge, ordering a bedstead, old mattresses, and sheets to be placed in the centre of the room. Fanny later recalled, 'every thing convinced me danger was hovering about me, & that this experiment could alone save me from its jaws.' So she climbed on the bed and Dubois placed a thin handkerchief over her face. Its transparency permitted her to see the seven men and nurse gather round the bed, but when she saw 'the glitter of polished Steel' she closed her eyes, unable to watch 'the terrible incision'. The experience was 'a terror that surpasses all description, & the most torturing pain', she wrote.

> When the dreadful steel was plunged into the breast—cutting through veins—arteries—flesh—nerves—I needed no injunctions not to restrain my cries. I began a scream that lasted unintermittingly during the whole time of the incision—& I almost marvel that it rings not in my Ears still! so excruciating was the agony. ... I then felt the Knife [rack]ling against the breast bone—scraping it! ... I bore it with all the courage I could exert, & never moved, nor stopt them, nor resisted, nor remonstrated, nor spoke ... When all was done, & they lifted me up that I might be put to bed ... I then saw my good Dr Larry, pale nearly as myself, his face streaked with blood, & his expression depicting grief, apprehension, & almost horrour.

Fanny recovered but it was six months before she could begin to record her ordeal. 'I dare not revise, nor read, the recollection is still so painful,' she wrote to her elder sister Esther.[1]

Fanny's account tells us clearly that operations were the last resort of surgeons and patients. Pain was not the only problem; the perils of blood loss and infection made all surgery life-threatening. Exposing a patient to such risks could only be justified when all other courses had been explored. When the diarist Samuel Pepys agreed to have his bladder stone removed in 1658, it was the only escape from 'a condition of constant and dangerous and most painful sickness and low condition and poverty'.[2] He knew he was fortunate to survive the operation: he preserved the stone in a special case and celebrated 'operation day' for the remainder of his life. And though anatomical knowledge and surgical techniques expanded considerably during the eighteenth and early nineteenth centuries, surgery remained a risky business. Major operations included amputation, hernia, ovariotomy, lithotomy (removal of bladder stones), trepan (cutting a hole in the skull to remove injured or diseased parts without disturbing the dura surrounding the brain), and many smaller procedures such as removing polyps or repairing fistula in the rectum. But most surgeons performed few operations. Records from Amsterdam suggest that on average, fewer than four lithotomies a year were performed between 1725 and 1821; a mortality rate of around 20 per cent indicates the risks involved. At large and prestigious London hospitals only a handful of major operations took place each month. University College hospital surgeon Robert Liston performed only two or three operations each month. Surgeon to the Royal Naval hospital in Plymouth, Stephen Hammick, undertook fewer than two amputations a month during his twenty-year career.

Because the risks of surgery were so high, an elaborate etiquette of medical consultations had developed. This was partly to ensure that patients were given every chance of alternative therapies: it also reassured surgeons that their decision to operate was sound. Larrey was not alone in reacting emotionally to Fanny's operation. Walking to the operating room was like 'going to a hanging', John Abernethy, surgeon at St Bartholomew's Hospital, told a friend: on occasion he was known to shed tears or vomit after a particularly terrible operation. Charles Bell spoke to his brother of 'anxious feelings' and 'indescribable anxiety'. His fellow surgeon at the Middlesex Hospital, James Arnott, described Bell's demeanour as 'the reluctance of one who has to face an unavoidable evil'.[3]

The problem of surgical pain had occupied surgeons over many centuries and led to various experiments. At the end of the eighteenth century, the London surgeon James Moore designed a heavy steel clamp which compressed the limb before amputation. His hope was that the pressure on the nerves might succeed in diminishing pain. But patients complained that the sensations this mechanism caused were as painful as the operation itself. In London in 1813 James Wardrop bled a particularly nervous young woman until she lost consciousness in order to remove a tumour from her head. The procedure was successful—Wardrop taught medical students the technique—but most surgeons considered it dangerous. They believed that an operation placed severe stress on the body's systems and understood pain as a vital stimulant which worked to protect the body during this risky time. Sometimes patients lost consciousness during operations because of the intense pain and blood loss—the condition was known as syncope. But to intentionally depress the body was believed to add to the inherent risks. The same argument limited the use of alcohol and opiates. Patients were often given a small dose either in advance or during an operation, but doping them to the point of unconsciousness was considered too risky. Nor did either drug succeed in calming the patient's mind, which for most surgeons was the key problem as the mind was the source of fears, anxieties, and emotions.

Had Fanny's doctors possessed a reliable method of pain relief we can be in no doubt that they would have offered it, and she would have taken it. Practitioners had always sought to relieve pain but within the classical medicine, developed in Greece in the fourth century BC, which dominated Western medicine until well into the nineteenth century, understandings of pain were very different from those we have today. In the classical view of the body, health and disease were understood to be determined by the balance of humours (fluids)—blood, phlegm, choler (yellow bile), and melancholy (black bile). These fulfilled specific life-giving functions within the body. Each person had a different and unique balance of these fluids which determined both constitution and personality. Physical appearance and temperament were explained by the predominant humour. A natural dominance of blood, say, produced a person with a red face and hasty temper; those with a natural excess of phlegm were pale-skinned and cool-natured. Amongst Chaucer's pilgrims in the *Canterbury Tales* we find the *sanguine* Franklin who revels in meat and wine, and the thin, *choleric* Reeve.

Health was enjoyed when the humours maintained their natural equilibrium and patients often sought advice from medical practitioners on appropriate regimes for achieving this. Imbalance in one of the vital fluids produced sickness and could be remedied by lifestyle—diet and exercise—or by therapies that restored the body to its natural balance. Excessive quantities of yellow bile produced inflammation; too much blood resulted in fever. Noxious or excess fluids could be drawn from the body through vomiting, bloodletting, or emetics. Humoralism encapsulated the whole person. No differentiation was made between physical or psychological symptoms; a physician would take as much account of the patient's state of mind as of a fever or rash. Medical consultations focused upon the individual patient. Specific diseases were described within medical theory, but both practitioners and patients believed strongly that health and sickness were individual experiences, distinct to particular bodies. Pain was believed to be a product of imbalance within the system and therapies like bloodletting were used in an attempt to draw the pain out of the body. It was taken to be a general indicator of ill-health and disease, rather than a specific entity which could be treated locally.

From the mid-seventeenth century onwards, the body's nervous system became a focus for new research into the physiology of nerves and muscles. The Swiss physician Albrecht von Haller distinguished between nerves (endowed with sensibility, an innate capacity to communicate sensations) and muscles (endowed with irritability, a kind of nervous power that resided in the muscles). Robert Whytt in Edinburgh confirmed that sensibility was located in the nerves and explained reflex as being caused by an unconscious sentient principle located in the spinal cord and brain which stimulated the muscles and caused movement. His work put a new stress on cerebral functions which was to prove crucial to understanding the later process of anaesthesia.

By the later eighteenth century, physicians like William Cullen, Professor at Edinburgh University, were convinced that the nervous system was pivotal to understanding health and sickness. 'Almost the whole of the diseases of the human body might be called NERVOUS,' proclaimed Cullen.[4] Sensibility was understood to vary by degrees in different people, according to the natural capacity of their nerves to receive and transmit sensations, and the irritability of their muscles. Imbalance of irritability, or excitement as it was called, became the new way of interpreting sickness. A certain degree of 'excitement' in the body was necessary for healthy functions; too little or too much put the body out of balance. Following the patterns of opposites established in humoral medicine, practitioners explained their treatment of sickness as a rebalancing of these dynamics. Depressants—bloodletting, emetics—restored health to patients suffering from excessive excitement. Stimulants like opiates or alcohol and 'shock' therapy using electricity returned excitement to a depleted body. Some patients lapped up these new ideas: 'I have no Fever at present, I have head-Ache, and Indigestion, & I have lately been convinc'd that I have Nerves,' wrote one sufferer.[5]

The new vogue for sensibility coloured the literature of the day, especially that of Laurence Sterne and Samuel Richardson. The prolific cast of characters filling the pages of *The Life and Opinions of Tristram Shandy* (1759–67) are absorbed by their engagement with the outside world. The view that feelings, rather than reason, should inform morals and social structures began to be expressed by philosophers and politicians. Scottish philosopher David Hume's moral, political, and literary essays, published in 1742, stressed how developing fine sensibilities lay at the root of self-improvement.

Man's judgement, he wrote, 'may be compared to a clock or watch, where the most ordinary machine is sufficient to tell the hours; but the most elaborate alone can point out the minutes and seconds, and distinguish the smallest differences of time'. A well-developed judgement meant that an individual 'feels too sensibly, how much all the rest of mankind fall short of the notions which he has entertained'.[6] As sensibility emerged as a yardstick of civilization, man's flesh and bones grew increasingly vulnerable to painful sensations.

From the mid-eighteenth century onwards, British use of opiates rose dramatically, suggesting a growing sensibility to pain. Doctors engaged with pain in a new way. For centuries, death had been viewed as a spiritual experience and the pains of the last hours or days of life were to be born in the expectation of divine redemption through eternal life. Patients' physical needs were cared for, but attention focused on confession and priestly absolution. As opiate use grew, so did the attendance of doctors at the bedsides of the dying. Opiates were part of a package of care; doctors also held patient's hands and uttered soothing words. Religion was not pushed away from the bedside; in fact medicine became its enabler. Pain relief gave patients a chance to resolve earthly matters without physical distractions. The Welsh physician John Jones's *The Mysteries of Opium Reveal'd* (1701) made no bones about its positive effects: 'causes a brisk, gay and good Humour ... Serenity, Alacrity, and Expediteness in Dispatching and Managing Business ... Ovation of the Spirits, Courage, Contempt of Danger ... takes away Grief, Fear, Anxieties, Peevishness, Fretfulness ... charms the Mind with Satisfaction, Acquiescence, Contentation, Equanimity, &c.' Commitment to the Divinely ordained suffering of childbirth also began to erode. Though not widely promoted—probably for fear of opposition, either real or imagined—some doctors began to use opiates in labour. But addiction to opiates was common. Toothache and neuralgia first prompted the Romantic poet Samuel Taylor Coleridge to take opium; he soon became dependent on its life-enhancing effects. Opium addiction cost him his marriage, severed his relationship with fellow poet William Wordsworth, and eventually contributed to his death. Thomas de Quincy's no-holds barred account of addiction, *The Confessions of an English Opium Eater* (1821), became a best-seller. Part of the attraction, of course, was opium's power of restoring youth and possibilities to the aging. It is impossible to determine whether the increased use of opiates was a cause or effect of a decreased social tolerance of pain. Nevertheless these fundamental schisms in old ideas of pain as functional and integral to healing spread through Europe. The Napoleonic wars give easy evidence of the strong political and military divide between France and England at the beginning of the nineteenth century, but the two nations shared a growing intolerance to pain: imports of opiates to France rose by 50 per cent between 1803 and 1807.

For Enlightenment optimists, medicine was crucial in the quest for perfectibility. Knowledge of disease and new therapies appeared to be powerful tools in the brave new world. The new gas chemistry, spearheaded in Britain by the political radical Joseph Priestley, promised revolutionary treatments. A mouse was the first to breathe the new kind of air, isolated by Priestley in 1774 and later called oxygen. Breathing the new air himself, Priestley noticed the effects on his chest: it felt 'particularly light and easy for some time afterwards'.[7] The dangers posed to health by 'bad air' from natural environments such as marshes or stagnant water had been stressed by Hippocrates centuries earlier. By the eighteenth century, air quality was high on the medical agenda. The army physician John Pringle considered outbreaks of fever epidemics and scurvy in soldiers' camps to be linked to the putrid air of the nearby marshes. Using Priestley's new breathable airs to cure disease was an obvious route to take. It fell to

Thomas Beddoes to test out this 'pneumatic medicine' which was to establish how gases had the power to transform bodily states.

Son of a well-to-do Shropshire tanner, Thomas Beddoes went to Oxford and then studied medicine in London and Edinburgh. He took up a chemistry post at Oxford and embraced the new French chemistry pioneered by Antoine Lavoisier that paralleled Priestley's work in researching the 'different kinds of air'. Fervent about the rights of man and the freedom to think independently, Beddoes developed close links with members of the Lunar Society of Birmingham including Joseph Priestley, Erasmus Darwin, Josiah Wedgewood, and James Watt. But after the French Revolution, when Britain went to war with France, known radicals were targeted by mobs. In 1791 during the Birmingham Riots, Priestley watched the destruction of his house, garden, and laboratory. Instruments were destroyed, books and manuscripts burnt: 'I afterwards heard that much pains were taken, but without effect, to get fire from my large electrical machine, which stood in the library,' he wrote.[8] Beddoes' own enlightened ideals were out of step for Oxford; he quit his post. Moving to Bristol in 1793, then a stronghold for political radicals, he sought to fulfil his dream that the new gases like oxygen could cure diseases like tuberculosis. Less than a year later Beddoes married Anna Edgeworth, daughter of Lunar friend Richard Lovell Edgeworth. The match surprised friends: Anna's cheerfulness, gaiety, and wit were the antithesis of Beddoes' fiery outspokenness. Nevertheless she engaged wholeheartedly with Beddoes' political and pamphleteering activities. Just as the Lunar circle had supported Priestley's researches with funding and equipment, so they mustered arms to launch Beddoes' dreams. On 21 March 1799 a notice in the *Bristol Gazette* announced a new medical institution that would treat incurable diseases like consumption, asthma, palsy, dropsy, and venereal conditions. It promised methods that were not painful, nor hazardous. The Pneumatic Institute was funded by subscriptions (mainly the Lunar circle) and offered free treatment. It became a honeypot to the Romantic poets Robert Southey and Samuel Taylor Coleridge, and radicals like Davies Giddy (later President of the Royal Society).

Pragmatically, Beddoes hoped to develop his methods by testing them on poor patients. Beddoes' rationale was developed through his own experience of respiring oxygen for several months: he lost weight, became flushed in the face, and suffered nosebleeds—typical characteristics of consumption. It seemed to him that excessive oxygen had caused the symptoms of consumption. Scurvy, he believed, was caused by too little oxygen. Rebalancing the components of the air in a body by respiring a particular gas seemed a logical way of restoring health. He recruited a young, untrained chemist to help run the Institute—Humphry Davy, later to become the most famous chemist of his generation. Beddoes was an 'uncommonly short and fat, [man] with little elegance of manners, and nothing characteristic externally of genius or science', Davy wrote to his mother after meeting his new employer.[9] Nevertheless the two men shared a conviction that chemistry was the source of life's powers and forces—Davy's earlier research into the nature of heat and light was built on that principle. One of the gases Davy researched as part of Beddoes' quest to discover a cure for a 'catalogue of diseases' was nitrous oxide.

Isolated by Joseph Priestley in the 1770s and called 'dephlogisticated nitrous air', nitrous oxide had been investigated by New York chemistry professor Samuel Mitchill: the 'gaseous oxyd of azote' was lethal if inhaled, suggested Mitchill. Davy's plan to investigate its composition, properties, and mode of operation on living beings was nothing less than audacious. After a succession of chemical experiments Davy turned to animals. How would nitrous oxide affect the nervous system; what were the differences between warm- and cold-blooded creatures? Through the process of respiration, he believed the gas would enter the blood and travel through the body. One lizard placed in a jar of nitrous oxide lay on his back with his paws resting on his belly 'seemingly dead', yet recovered when placed in shallow water. Davy observed that this lifeless state was preceded by a period of intense activity in the creature. This sequence of stimulation followed by depression was also seen in rabbits, mice, fish, flies, snails, and earthworms. Reassured that nitrous oxide did not cause instant death, Davy breathed it himself: 'I was aware of the danger,' he wrote, anticipating that he might feel painful or depressing sensations. On the first occasion he felt intoxicated and his pulse increased. The next day he breathed again and this time he experienced the gas's 'extraordinary powers of action'. He felt a gentle pressure on his muscles and a 'highly pleasurable thrilling' extended across his chest and extremities, he said. Under its influence a world of subdued hues was cast into dazzling technicolour. His hearing became more acute, 'the thrilling increased, the sense of muscular power became greater, and at last an irresistible propensity to action was indulged in', he recorded. From this point Davy was utterly absorbed by nitrous oxide. He breathed different quantities for different lengths of time and at different times of the day, on each occasion noting the effects on his pulse, sleeping, and senses. He tried it after consuming a bottle of wine, before eating, and after eating. Sometimes he breathed the gas three or four times on the same day. He noticed it relieved minor aches and pains. On the most memorable occasions he experienced 'sublime emotions connected with highly vivid ideas'.[10] Friends and visitors to the Institute were urged to participate in this new world. Rather than revolutionizing medical treatments, nitrous oxide revolutionized individual sensibilities by producing: 'a delirium of pleasurable sensations', enthused Robert Southey after breathing the gas.[11]

The sensations of nitrous oxide fanned the self-interest of Enlightenment figures but capturing the experience in words proved almost impossible. How can such 'new and particular sensations' be expressed in the confines of existing vocabulary, mused word-lover James Thomson, later to write the thesaurus. Even sceptics like Josiah Wedgwood were captivated by its powers: he experienced the 'most singular sensations' which made him feel 'lighter than the atmosphere', as if he were about to 'mount to the top of the room', he wrote.[12] Some found themselves on the fringes of addiction: 'I went on breathing with great vehemence, not from a difficulty of inspiration, but from an eager avidity for more air,' affirmed J. Tobin. Stephen Hammick refused to let Davy take the bag away, so pleasurable was the feeling.[13] Just seeing the bag caused Davy to desire the gas.

Opium addiction was a problem of the times and addicts found it brought dreadful depressions in its wake. Nitrous oxide left no such dark legacy but recollections of 'more unmingled pleasure than I had ever before experienced', wrote opium user Samuel Taylor Coleridge.[14] That a chemical had the power to intensify engagement with the natural world harmonized with Enlightenment philosophies. But the nitrous oxide experiments brought no therapeutic breakthroughs. The conservative outcry against the French Revolution and all things French tarred gas chemistry and other radical pursuits such as mesmerism—later tried as a method of surgical pain relief—as subversive and dangerous. Davy sensed this shift and in the last few pages of his work on nitrous oxide, written in June 1800, he noted disconsolately that the common theory of excitability 'is most probably founded on a false generalisation' as variations of diseased action may be 'infinite and specific in different organs' and thus beyond the power of agents which acted on the whole system.[15]

The Pneumatic Institute was of its moment. Davy left to follow his star at the Royal Institution; a typhus epidemic hit Bristol, and Beddoes became caught up in treating its victims. Afterwards Beddoes restructured the Institute into a Preventive Institution to help the sick poor. Gas chemistry, the hoped-for panacea, lost its appeal in the cool light of a conservative dawn.

Davy's work plays an important role within the history of anaesthesia. He proved that gases could change bodily states. But we should not be surprised that Davy did not leap upon nitrous oxide as a potential anaesthetic: he was a product of eighteenth-century bodily understandings. The possibility of suspending sensation without endangering life could not be imagined within the 1790s' configurations of the nervous system: the associations and interdependence between sensibility and irritability were too complex to disentangle. Pain was thought integral to the body's functions, and essential to healing. Davy thought it possible that sensation could outlive all other powers of the body: his greatest fear was of being buried alive and he exacted a promise from his brother that upon Davy's death, there would be a ten-day period of grace before burial. There is no doubt that Davy would have applied the powers of nitrous oxide to surgery had he thought this plausible. His suggestion that the gas might play a role in surgical operations where there was minimal blood loss was made on the basis of its stimulatory characteristics. It would be equivalent to small quantities of opiates or alcohol found to be helpful in reviving patients debilitated from the stress of an operation. But although physiology offered no solution to the problem of pain, the philosophies underpinning its role in society had begun to shift.

In Christian theology, pain entered the world after Eve's disobedience in the Garden of Eden and remained central to humanity. Over the centuries, mankind sought to alleviate physical suffering yet also accepted its inevitability. But during the eighteenth century there was a key shift in both social and medical attitudes to pain. A new attention to feeling and alleviation of painful sensations crept in on the back of Enlightenment philosophies and spread through Europe. The radical realignment placed sensibility as the crux of moral behaviour and drove a raft of reforms focusing on particularly vulnerable groups: slaves, animals, prisoners, and children. It was underpinned by the new physiology which viewed the nervous system as the body's primary interface with the outside world. In England, the 1780s marked the beginning of the campaign by William Wilberforce and his associates to abolish the Slave Trade: in the Austrian Empire, Joseph II, brother of Marie-Antoinette, abolished serfdom and the death penalty. Sensibility equated to civilization: 'Am I not a man and a brother?' asked the black slave depicted on the yellow jasper medallion manufactured by Josiah Wedgwood for the Society for the Suppression of the Slave Trade. The new awareness that all races experienced pain (though some less than others) also extended to animals. England was notorious for its violent and bloody sports. Bull, dog, and bearbaiting, cock-fighting, and boxing had entertained generations on feast and fair days since medieval times. Some observers like the seventeenth-century diarist John Evelyn disliked the 'barbarous cruelties' of such sports. Once when passing the main London bear-garden, Paris Garden in Bankside, Southwark, Evelyn saw a bull toss a dog so high in the air it landed on the lap of a lady sitting in a box above the arena. The Puritans attempted to stop bearbaiting, though in his *History of England*, Thomas Babington Macaulay suggested that this was not on account of the pain caused to the bear, but rather the pleasure given to the spectator.

The moral philosophy upon which the shift against cruelty to animals was built may seem natural to us: that animals, as well as humans, have an innate capacity to experience pain. Thus, every *body*, be it of man, mammal, or insect, operated within the same dynamic framework of anatomy and physiology and was vulnerable to suffering from unpleasant physical sensations. But it challenged long-held views about man's superiority on the basis of his reason, speech, and soul. The Church of England clergyman Humphry Primatt was one of the first to express views about animals: 'pain is pain, whether it be inflicted on man or on beast; and the creature that suffers it, whether man or beast, being sensible of the misery of it while it lasts, suffers evil,' he wrote in *A Dissertation on the Duty of Mercy and the Sin of Cruelty to Brute Animals* (1776). Primatt supported his arguments with many references to the Bible: neither colour nor species justified the enslavement or tyranny of other living beings. Sensibility was common to all. Animals, noted Primatt, are 'no less sensible of pain than a man. He has similar nerves and organs of sensation.' Primatt's views spread.

The Dorset clergyman John Toogood appended part of Primatt's text to his sermon published in the 1790s. Promoted as a 'Shrovetide gift to his parishioners', Toogood was no doubt trying to refocus the long history of animal baiting on feast days. Primatt's arguments underpinned later debates on animals and pain. The moral question about animals, wrote the philosopher Jeremy Bentham in his *Introduction to the Principles of Morals and Legislation* (1789), 'is not, Can they reason?, nor Can they talk? but, Can they suffer? Why should the law refuse its protection to any sensitive being? The time will come when humanity will extend its mantle over everything which breathes.' For Bentham, sensation was the key to determining both moral behaviour and legislation:

> Nature has placed mankind under the governance of two sovereign masters, pain and pleasure. It is for them alone to point out what we ought to do, as well as to determine what we shall do. On the one hand the standard of right and wrong, on the other the chain of causes and effects, are fastened to their throne. They govern us in all we do, in all we say, in all we think.

Child of the Enlightenment, Bentham drew on the philosophies of John Locke and David Hume amongst many others. He also acknowledged his debt to Joseph Priestley with whom he had corresponded on chemical experiments: 'Priestley was the first ... who taught my lips to pronounce this sacred truth:—That the greatest happiness of the greatest number is the foundation of morals and legislation.' Bentham's felicific calculus became a powerful influence on nineteenth-century conceptions of liberty and the state developed by the philosopher John Stuart Mill among others.

From the 1800s new research into the brain's anatomy and physiology started to reshape old understandings of sensation. Work by the British physician Charles Bell and French physiologist Francois Magendie in the 1810s established that different parts of the brain were responsible for specific functions and showed how sensations and movement were carried by different nerves. Another Frenchman, Marie Jean-Pierre Flourens, performed a series of experiments on pigeons in 1824 which demonstrated the specificity of functions. When a pigeon lost both cerebral hemispheres it became blind; losing only one hemisphere caused blindness in the opposite eye. The idea that bodily functions could be specifically located within the brain, and that processes like respiration and circulation could operate independently, later became the basis for the science developed around the anaesthetic process. But at this point, the knowledge that sensations were controlled by nerve centres in the brain, rather than the spinal cord, caused some surgeons to think differently about the pain of surgery.

'There is not an individual who does not shudder at the idea of an operation, however skilful the surgeon or urgent the case, knowing the great pain that the patient must endure,' wrote Henry Hill Hickman, a Shropshire surgeon, who published his ideas on suspended animation in 1824.[16] Suspended animation was thought to be a form of asphyxia, a shortage of oxygen. Although it was recognized as a state very close to death, since the late eighteenth century doctors had used resuscitation techniques to restore life in such circumstances. Prompted by a heartfelt desire to relieve both the anticipation and actual suffering of a severe operation, Hickman tested out his hypothesis that the 'torpid state' produced by inhaling carbon dioxide gas offered a useful interlude of insensibility. Puppies, rabbits, and mice were placed in the gas until respiration ceased; Hickman removed legs, ears, or tails, and dressed wounds; the animals gradually recovered consciousness. He took careful note of bleeding and the speed of healing but the most impressive fact was the apparent absence of suffering whilst he was using the knife. Hickman had no links to the medical bigwigs of the day but he did know Thomas Andrew Knight, Fellow of the Royal Society, who lived nearby in Downton Castle. Knight was renowned locally for his prize-winning Merino-Ryland crossbred sheep, and further afield for his expertise in plant and vegetable physiology. Hickman wrote to Knight describing his experiments and then printed a small pamphlet. We may expect this to have caused a stir. In fact Hickman's proposals fell on stony ground. Hickman persisted. In 1828 he travelled to France and urged King Charles X to consider his work. It was discussed at the Académie Royale de Médicine, and Fanny Burney's surgeon, Larrey, thought it of interest. But nothing came of it. Eventually Hickman returned to England and died in 1830, aged only 31. Not only did Hickman's ideas challenge the essential purpose of pain, but suspending consciousness and respiration by inhaling a lethal gas seemed to skate too close to death.

Carbon dioxide had been identified in the 1750s through Joseph Black's research into different kinds of air. Miners were familiar with the 'bad' air at the bottom of shafts and one of the best-known natural occurrences of carbon dioxide was on the outskirts of Naples, near Lake Agano, once the crater of a volcano. 'On its bare and melancholy shores we found the celebrated Grotto del Cane,' noted L. Simond, who visited the area in 1818.[17] The Grotto received its name from the unfortunate dogs placed into the cave to demonstrate for visitors the effects of the gas. To those not au fait with new understandings of physiology it seemed as if magic. One visitor wrote that the dog

> presently loses all motion, falls down as dead or in a swoon; the limbs convulsed and trembling, till at last no more signs of life appear than a very weak and almost insensible beating of the heart and arteries, which if the animal be left a little longer, quickly ceases too ... But if it is taken out in time, and laid in the open air, it soon comes to life again.[18]

The Grotto was still listed in the 1893 edition of Baedeker's Italian guidebook.

Carbon dioxide aroused geographical and scientific interest but for fun and frolics nitrous oxide's alter ego—laughing gas—proved a better bet. The Adelphi Theatre in the Strand—'home of melodrama and screaming farce', claimed one London directory—staged Monsieur Henry's show in the 1820s. The playbill promised instruction through 'novel and interesting experiments on gas' and 'peals of laughter' provoked by the 'wonderful effects' of the gas.[19] It was a curious mishmash of chemistry and farce. Christian Schoenbein, a

German-Swiss chemist who later discovered gun-cotton and ozone, described how the curtain rose to reveal a semi-circle of large rubber bladders with glinting metal taps. M. Henry gave a short description of the gas and its properties: 'in a way which would have done credit to a professor of chemistry', noted Schoenbein. Then the fun began. The first volunteer was booed off the stage by the audience, as was the second. M. Henry asked for cooperation. The next volunteer sat in a chair and inhaled the gas. When the bladder was removed, he continued to sit holding his nose, causing roars of laughter; then he leapt and bounded around the stage. But the audience's interest waned: 'All nonsense and humbug!', they began to cry. M. Henry asked the sceptic who began the revolt to come and try the gas. After emptying the largest bladder of gas he 'beat around' M. Henry 'like a madman' and assaulted him. Schoebein had tried laughing gas himself whilst staying with one of his friends who was an amateur chemist. After making large quantities of the gas, they invited friends to join them in the garden and inhale. One visitor, sceptical about the gas's powers, breathed a lot: 'he began to dance and devastate the adjoining flower-bed in his ecstasy,' remembered Schoebein. It was, he thought, a strong contender to replace champagne at the end of dinner parties.[20] Singing about laughing gas could be as entertaining as breathing it. Published around 1830, 'Laughing Gas, a new comic song, sung with unbounded Applause', by Mr W. Smith of the Royal Surrey Theatre, extolled the tribulations of 'Poor Jeremy Jones' who 'swallowed a bladder of laughing gas', in eleven verses. Nor were such pastimes unique to the British temperament.

Across the Atlantic, advertisements promised crowds more laughter than they had had in the previous six months if they visited the Grand Exhibition 'of the effects produced by inhaling Nitrous Oxid, Exhilarating or Laughing Gas!', demonstrated by Gardner

Quincy Colton. No longer able to afford to continue at medical school, Colton lectured on popular scientific subjects. His shows attracted thousands of visitors and the one held on 10 December 1844 in Hartford proved particularly interesting. One of the young men who breathed the gas came strongly under its influence: running and jumping he bruised his legs so badly on a wooden bench they began to bleed. Observing these antics was Horace Wells, a local dentist. Wells asked Colton to help him try an experiment: Wells breathed nitrous oxide and had a tooth removed. Colton taught him how to make the gas and went on his way. Using a bladder and a wooden tube, Wells succeeded in giving nitrous oxide to a handful of patients during tooth extractions. He was convinced he had discovered a major technique and set up a demonstration on a man having a tooth extracted at Boston's elite Massachusetts General Hospital. Disaster. In front of a large audience the man complained he felt pain: 'the whole was denounced as an imposition and no-one was inclined to assist me in further experiments,' said Wells. On reflection he realized that nerves had got the better of him; the gasbag had been removed too soon. Wells was given no second chance. The intense disappointment of failure 'brought on an illness from which I did not recover for many months', he later recalled.[21] Wells is a tragic hero: he missed out on the discovery of nitrous oxide anaesthesia by a whisker. By the time he was credited for his work it was too late: he had committed suicide.

We may imagine that after Wells's failure with nitrous oxide, ether anaesthesia was waiting in the wings. In fact there was no such view. Many surgeons believed pain relief was an unachievable quest: 'a chimera that we can no longer pursue in our times', asserted New York surgeon Valentine Mott.[22] He, and many others, ignored the potential of mesmerism. An early form of hypnosis, mesmerism was introduced by Anton Mesmer in the 1790s. It was, he explained, 'a fluid universally diffused … the medium of a mutual influence between the heavenly bodies'.[23] Like laughing gas, mesmerism was popularized at fairs and exhibitions. It was also tried in surgery. The French surgeon Jules Cloquet successfully performed a mastectomy using 'hypnotic analgesia' in 1829. More successes followed, promoted in England in the 1830s by John Elliotson, Professor of Medicine at University College Hospital, and publicized in the *Zoist*. But mesmerism could not be explained by contemporary science: it was tainted by its mysterious history. Most doctors considered it a sham: 'the girls who are magnetised deceive and cheat. They pretend to read with the back of their head, and prophecy all sorts of stuff,' complained the President of the Royal College of Surgeons, Benjamin Brodie.[24] A few doctors pursued mesmeric anaesthesia but not many managed to make it work. James Esdaile, a Scottish surgeon working in India, reported over a thousand successful operations carried out in the mid-1840s on patients rendered insensible to the pain through mesmerism: introducing mesmerism to the London hospitals was his vision. It remained unfulfilled.

Only twelve months after Wells failed to prove nitrous oxide's anaesthetic powers at Massachusetts General Hospital, fellow dentist William Thomas Green Morton succeeded in establishing ether and began anaesthesia as we know it today. What made Morton succeed? Partly personality and partly chemistry accounted for his success. Morton was not alone in experimenting with ether. In the southern state of Georgia, a country doctor in a small agricultural community, Crawford Long, had operated under ether in the early 1840s. In Jefferson, as elsewhere, local youths entertained themselves with laughing gas. But Long could not manufacture it: he offered them ether instead. First synthesized in the sixteenth century by Valerius Cordus and sold by chemists as 'sweet vitriol', ether was used as a stimulant and anti-spasmodic; it could be inhaled or swallowed.

Ether frolics became a local novelty. When James Venables, one of the young ether sniffers, needed a minor operation for the removal of a cyst but was terrified of pain, Long thought of using ether. 'Breathe ether, then I'll cut off the cyst,' he advised Venables. Success. Venables only believed what had happened when Long showed him the cyst. Long continued the practice on one or two patients a year. But he never reported his results because he could not satisfy himself as to whether the anaesthetic effects had been produced by the ether, or the patient's imagination. Nor was there much praise for Long's innovation locally: most of the community were devout Christians who believed it was against God's will to avoid physical pain. Ether breathing was as much a moral as physical risk.

Morton's success was driven by business ambitions, rather than sympathy for patients. By the 1840s, dental technology was capable of producing good sets of artificial teeth that looked vastly superior to earlier designs. Yet a good fit relied on extracting all the decayed stumps and roots of original teeth from the jaw, and often patients could not bear the pain.

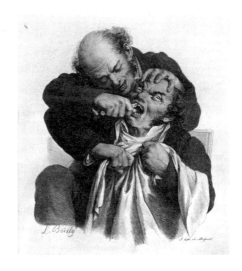

Figure 1 Many patients, partcularly females could not endure the pain of tooth extractions. Coloured litho c.1826.

Some patients tried to fortify themselves by having a glass or two of wine; some ran away in the middle of the extractions. It was this un-tapped market that stimulated Morton's researches: the surefire way to boost dental profits was to solve the problem of pain. He quizzed his landlord and fellow dentist, Charles T. Jackson, on the charac-teristics of ether: Jackson used ether as 'toothache drops'. Morton borrowed Jackson's chemistry textbooks to bone up on ether: 'there was nothing new or particularly dangerous in the inhaling of ether,' he reassured himself.[25] After establishing that sulphuric ether was the most effective form of the chemical, Morton tried it on animals, then he inhaled ether from a handkerchief and lost consciousness. On coming round, 'I felt a numbness in my limbs, with a sensa-tion like nightmare ... Gradually, I regained power over my limbs, and full consciousness ... I had been insensible between seven and eight minutes,' he said.[26] On 30 September 1846 fortune struck. A young man, Eben Frost, called on Morton in the evening in great pain, desperate to have a tooth extracted. 'Could it be done using mesmerism to avoid pain?', he asked Morton. 'I have something better,' promised Morton. From all accounts it was a success: Frost declared himself 'perfectly well and enraptured with the novelty and successful result of the experiment'.[27] Morton was spurred on: he persuaded Chief Surgeon John Collins Warren at Massachusetts General Hospital to let him demonstrate the remarkable powers of his discovery; he also visited Commissioner of Patents R. H. Eddy, keen to secure his legal rights.

On the morning of Friday 16 October Morton arrived at Mas-sachusetts General Hospital, accompanied by Eben Frost, living proof of the discovery. They arrived late: Morton had been delayed by the last-minute adjustments to his apparatus. But whereas the drama of the situation had terrified Wells, Morton's showmanship won through. Edward Abbott, 20 years old, was sitting in a chair, waiting to have a tumour on the left side of jaw removed. Morton took him by the hand, told him that the new preparation would ease some, if not all of the pain, pointed out Eben Frost and asked, 'Are you afraid?' 'No,' replied Abbott, 'I feel confident that you will do precisely as you tell me.' Once Abbott became insensible, Morton signalled to Warren to begin the operation. Warren, greatly surprised that Abbott did not start or cry during the incision, removed the tumour. During the last part Abbott moved his limbs and cried out a little, Warren was dubious about the success until he quizzed Abbott on his experience. Abbott was adamant that he had not felt pain: the incision, he said, was like a 'blunt instrument passed roughly across his neck'.

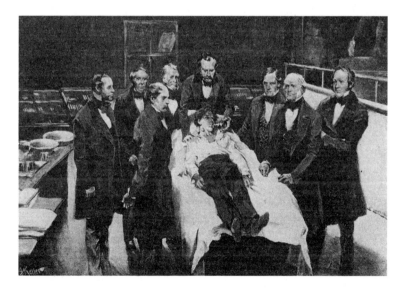

Figure 2 William Morton's demonstration of ether at Massachusetts General Hospital on 16 October 1846, painted fifty years or so after the event. The artist depicts Abbott lying down rather than sitting in a chair.

The following day a further successful operation was performed without the patient suffering pain. To be sure, luck was on Morton's side. Ether produced anaesthetic effects more reliably than nitrous oxide—had Wells chosen ether things may have been different—and there was no suggestion that any of Morton's patients suffered breathing difficulties during inhalations. Warren and the other surgeons endorsed Morton's discovery, and the Boston community began to buzz with excitement. But very soon clouds appeared in the sky.

When Jackson learnt of Morton's plan to patent ether he convinced Eddy he should also share in any financial return from ether as it was he who gave Morton the idea. A compromise was reached and Jackson and Morton submitted a patent application to the US Patent Office on 27 October 1846. Then war broke out. Boston dentists published a manifesto protesting against Morton's actions; hospital surgeons stopped using the preparation, partly because Morton would not reveal its identity, and partly because of the patent protections. Morton backtracked. He gave surgeons at the hospital an inhaler and agreed to reveal the identity of his preparation, providing they kept it secret: it was given the name 'Letheon'. On 7 November 1846 surgeons began using ether again and a couple of days later at the Boston Society of Medical Improvement, Henry J. Bigelow, a surgeon at the hospital, gave a paper on the new phenomenon. It was controversial, he said, for Morton to be patenting 'an agent capable of mitigating human suffering' and tried to explain the reasons. Its use should be restricted in case of hazards, and dentists were accustomed to working with secret processes. There was no doubt, he concluded, that the new preparation 'promised to be one of the most important discoveries of the age'.[28] Morton's attempt to patent his discovery and reap financial profit was not unusual within dentistry. Dental practitioners regularly sought to patent new mechanical inventions and Morton had a history of shady business ventures. Suffering pain during operations had been a tribulation of humankind for centuries: Morton could have visualized himself as the world's benefactor but probably even he did not envisage the way in which anaesthesia would be taken up. His vision was of the material return from his discovery.

On 12 November 1846 Jackson and Morton were issued with the Letter Patent No. 4848 but this compounded rather than resolved the difficulties. Wells, encouraged by friends, attempted to set the record straight and in a letter to the editor of the *Hartford Courant* wrote:

> If Drs Jackson and Morton claim something else, I reply that it is the same in principle, if not in name, and they can not use anything which will produce more satisfactory results, and I made these results known to both these individuals, more than a year since. After making the above statement of facts, I leave it for the public to decide to whom belongs the honor of discovery.[29]

Jackson sent an account of ether to the Académie des Sciences in Paris, claiming ownership of the discovery. The wrangle over priority of discovery lasted many years. Neither Morton, Jackson, or Wells ever received any kind of financial benefit for their part in the discovery of anaesthesia. Wells committed suicide in 1848; Morton died in 1868, still waging war with Jackson over their part in the discovery of anaesthesia.

But in December 1846 this was all to come. Boston surgeons were gaining confidence in ether but its future remained precarious. Many practical and intellectual controversies would have to be resolved before anaesthesia became routine in surgery. First, ether had to woo Europe.

2

. . . .

DISCOVERIES

Cunard's dock in Boston harbour on 3 December 1846: the final mail was loaded on board the paddle steamer *Acadia,* and she set sail, stopping briefly at Halifax for fuel and passengers before continuing to Liverpool. Few were aware of the momentous news carried in letters aboard the ship. Enthralled by William Morton's convincing demonstration of anaesthesia in Massachusetts General Hospital on 16 October, the Boston medical community had spent the past six weeks experimenting with ether. Now, word of the discovery was being sent to Britain.

Atlantic seas were stormy but the *Acadia*—one of the four ships which inaugurated Samuel Cunard's transatlantic steamship services in 1840—took just thirteen days to reach England, docking in Liverpool on 16 December. The Boston discovery must have been the talk of the deck, or the saloon: within forty-eight hours ether was mentioned in the *Liverpool Mercury.* The ship's surgeon, William Fraser, certainly knew of ether for he departed swiftly to his home town of Dumfries where his friend and surgeon William Scott later gave it to a young man who had suffered a compound fracture of his thigh in a railway accident. Meanwhile, news of ether was travelling south to London, to the home of American botanist Francis Boott.

Renowned worldwide for his botanic skills—his collection of North American plants was housed at the Royal Botanic Gardens at Kew—Boott had settled in London in 1820 and became part of the metropolis's cultural elite, joining the Linnean and Athenaeum Clubs. His links to Boston remained strong, fuelled by close friendships to men like Jacob Bigelow. Boott and Bigelow had bonded many years previously during an expedition to the White Mountains of New Hampshire. Bigelow, also an authority on botany, had become Professor of Materia Medica at Harvard University—a subject closely linked to botany as at that time most drugs were derived from plant material. Bigelow and his son, Henry, surgeon at Massachusetts General Hospital, had watched Morton's demonstration of ether. Henry subsequently performed several operations under ether and in November, Jacob took his daughter, Mary, to have a tooth extracted under ether by Morton himself. Jacob watched Mary inhale for about a minute, then fall asleep. She did not flinch during the extraction and woke with no remembrance of pain. This clinched Jacob's view that he had witnessed what promised to be 'one of the most important discoveries' of the age: he picked up his pen and wrote to his old friend.

Opening his mail at his home in Gower Street, London, on 17 December, Boott read Bigelow's account: 'limbs and breasts have been amputated, arteries tied, tumours extirpated, and many hundreds of teeth extracted, without … the least pain.' Mary's experience was 'an entire illusion'.[30] Boott immediately recognized the portent of Bigelow's news: he wrote to James Robinson, a dentist who lived in the same street; to Robert Liston, Professor of Surgery at University College Hospital, widely acknowledged to be London's finest surgeon; and to the *Lancet*. The idea that ether could solve the problem of dental and surgical pain galvanized Robinson and Liston. Robinson, a tempestuous character who had been at the forefront of establishing dentistry as a profession rather than a trade, set about devising an apparatus. On 19 December in front of Boott and his family, Robinson extracted 'a firmly fixed molar tooth' from Miss Lonsdale 'without the least sense of pain, or the movement of a muscle'. He tried the process on other patients—but failed to produce insensibility. 'I attribute the failure to the defect in the valve of the mouthpiece,' said Boott—Robinson went back to the drawing board.[31] Liston also watched Robinson's administration. Then he visited Peter Squire, pharmacist to Queen Victoria and president of the Royal Pharmaceutical Society, to order his own apparatus. (Squire's nephew was William Squire, Liston's medical student.) Squire 'hastily' put together an apparatus for Liston and on 21 December ether was tried at University College Hospital. 'Gentlemen! this Yankee dodge beats mesmerism hollow,' Liston reputedly declared to onlookers after amputating the leg of his patient, Frederick Churchill. Like Abbott in Boston, Churchill had moaned and stirred during the operation. Nevertheless Liston was convinced of ether's potential: it had 'the most perfect and satisfactory results' and was 'a fine thing for operating surgeons', he wrote to Boott that evening.[32] Then he hosted a celebratory dinner party at which he demonstrated the effects of ether on one of the guests.

Over Christmas, one of Liston's former students James Young Simpson, now a popular Edinburgh physician, travelled to London to hear the news of ether firsthand. But Liston's Christmas cheer was short-lived. Returning to work on 1 January 1847, Liston watched his patient, hoping to have his arm amputated without pain, inhale ether for ten minutes without success. Three days later, a woman about to have a breast tumour removed inhaled the vapour for more than twenty minutes without any effect. Liston was infuriated and sent for Robinson and his redesigned inhaler. Fortunately Robinson had simply to cross the road to the hospital: within minutes the patient was unconscious.

Etherization, ethereal inhalation, ethereal narcotism: a multiplicity of terms was used to describe the new process of breathing ether. The American physician and poet Oliver Wendell Holmes had advised Morton to name the state produced by ether: 'I would have a name pretty soon, and consult some accomplished scholar, such as President Everett or Dr Bigelow, senior, before fixing upon the terms, which will be repeated by the tongues of every civilized race of mankind,' Holmes wrote in November 1846.[33] Morton took up Holmes's suggestion—anaesthesia—though it did not come into general use for several years. But whatever the descriptive used, news of ether's power to remove surgical pain was travelling the world. In France, a 'commission for ether' was established by its Académies of sciences and medicine. Louis Velpeau, Professor of Clinical Surgery, was initially cautious, and then won over by ether's effects: 'surgery will gain benefits, wonderful benefits from the inhalations of ether during surgical operations,' he enthused.[34] In Austria's Imperial Stables, several stallions were castrated under ether watched by the Lord High Master of the Horse, Count Julius von Hellingshausen. A young surgeon in Berlin, Rudlof Virchow, later to become famous for his work on cellular pathology, experienced 'excellent results' with ether and Johann Langenbeck of Gottingen proclaimed that 'unlike many other acclaimed innovations which prove two-day wonders, this will prove a lasting blessing'.[35] Across Europe, doctors agreed that ether's powers were amazing: though its inconsistencies were perturbing, and its risks terrifying.

Much of the medical concern for the risks of ether hailed from its history. Classified as a narcotic and a poison in pharmacopoeias, ether was a popular chemical for demonstrations in medical schools. Students watched it stimulate, comatize, and eventually kill animals. Was the state of lethargy and coma produced by ether simply a form of asphyxia, or was it a new bodily state? Few had answers. The *London Medical Gazette* warned that ether 'must be regarded as producing a state of poisoning in which the nervous system is most powerfully affected'.[36]

Doctors were presented with a difficult dilemma. 'I could not try ether on my rich patients for my sake, nor on the poor for their sake,' one Dublin doctor later told Simpson. One solution was for doctors to try it on themselves, or each other. Nottinghamshire physician Dr Gill breathed ether whilst his friends gathered round, pinching his fingers and passing a needle through his skin to check for sensibility. Medical caution frustrated some patients. When Miss B inhaled ether the dentist, unsure about her state of sensibility, did not extract her teeth. She was greatly disappointed on recovering and insisted on inhaling ether again. This time she screamed during each extraction, but awoke saying she had felt no pain.

Patients responded in very different ways. Some became as insensible as breathing corpses—and as close to death. Others grew excited and lost their sense of propriety: 'Now we'll dance the Polka—Now we'll dance the Polka,' a respectable solicitor proposed to Robinson on regaining consciousness. A clergyman kept his eyes open under ether and 'appeared perfectly conscious of what was going on around him'. We 'certainly thought it was a failure', said Robinson. Yet the clergyman astounded him, exclaiming, 'I would not have believed it! I have lost my tooth! But how or when I know not, I never felt it.'[37] Patients were entranced by ether's effects. A middle-aged woman breathed the vapour at Westminster Hospital: her lower limbs twitched whilst tumours were removed from her labia, but she felt no pain. She awoke confused and disorientated, unable to believe the operation had taken place and cried from 'the combined result of apprehension, wonder, and delight'.[38] In the Edinburgh Royal Infirmary, James Miller removed some dead bone from the leg of an Irish workman. 'I suppose you won't let me operate today?', he said to the patient at the conclusion. 'Certainly not', retorted the patient, 'I must be asleep; we can try it another time.' Only the laughter and applause of the onlookers persuaded the Irishman that ether had saved him from suffering. His delight was such that he refused to leave the table until he had shared the 'strange medley of imaginary fights and killings going on around him' that had been his experience of 'going under'.[39]

But ether did not work on some patients. At St Thomas' Hospital, breathing the vapour caused a strong fit man to cough so much and become purple in the face that doctors withdrew it, for fear of it causing congestion in the brain and the lungs, although the next patient became perfectly insensible within minutes. Such discrepancies were puzzling. What were the exact principles for successful ether administration? surgeon dentist Chitty Clendon, exasperated by his failures, demanded of the *Lancet*. Across the Channel, the French surgeon Boullay echoed his despair: 'No one has yet determined even the proper dose of ether to be given.'[40] During early January 1847 many doctors were trialling ether and experimenting with different types of inhalers and face-pieces, amending and altering features as they went along. Robinson and Squire had had to re-design their inhalers within a very short space of time. Andrew Ure, member of the Pharmaceutical Society, suggested 'a hood to enclose the head' with 'a glass window in front'. At Bristol General Hospital, perhaps in memory of Davy's technique for breathing nitrous oxide, ether was given in a pig's bladder, and in Edinburgh, Professor James Miller abandoned all apparatus in favour of a 'bell-shaped sponge' which was saturated in ether and placed over the patient's nose and mouth. Each inventor was like a fond parent, seeing 'advantages in his own offspring which he failed to find in that of others', said a report

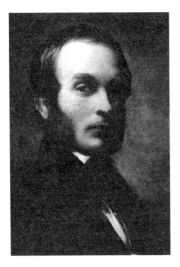

Figure 3 Portrait of John Snow by Thomas Jones Barker, painted in advance of his emergence as London's first anaesthetist and exhibited at the Royal Academy of Art in May 1847.

from the Pharmaceutical Society. Few methods seemed foolproof. The take-up of ether, particularly in London, may have remained patchy had it not been for the work of a Soho general practitioner, John Snow.

Snow's origins were humble: first son of a Yorkshire labourer, he had served his medical apprenticeship in Newcastle upon Tyne and then worked as an assistant to provincial general practitioners. Since arriving in London in 1836 and gaining his qualifications, Snow had slowly but painstakingly dug a niche for himself in the competitive and elitist London medical networks. He was a master of the new scientific view of the body which had emerged at the beginning of the nineteenth century: that the human body was constructed of organs and systems which had universal and predictable functions, and that disease was specific and local. Although he was respected by many for his forthright and unequivocal application of the new medicine, Snow's efforts were not reflected in profits. He attended a small, but loyal group of patients, most of whom lived in his locality of Soho. For the most part, this meant attending births, visiting the sick, often thrice daily, and prescribing remedies. Ether was to change this, perhaps more rapidly than he could ever have anticipated.

The striking thing about Snow is that despite his lowly background and Yorkshire vowels which set him apart from most London doctors, he was particularly well placed to exploit ether's potential. He had a strong interest in the chemistry and physiology of respiration and inhaled gases. In the early 1840s he had researched asphyxia and considered the effects of different 'volatile medicines' (one of which was ether) on the mechanism of respiration. He noted how in the lungs, ether separated from the blood and escaped with the breath 'in the gaseous form with the carbonic acid gas and watery vapour'.[41] These effects could be beneficial in certain cases of lung disease, he concluded. He had also developed a pump for resuscitating stillborn babies. This grounding in the new science, a strong belief that pain served no purpose, and, at the most down to earth level, a struggle to make a decent living combined to create a rare mixture of skills and motivation. Among the first to watch Robinson administer ether, Snow was captivated from the start. But unlike most doctors who obtained ether and sought a willing patient, Snow obtained ether and began a series of chemical and physiological experiments.

Snow's New Year of 1847 began with a flurry of experimental work in his rooms at 54 Frith Street, Soho. His conviction that scientific principles should form the basis of medical practice drove his research. The first questions he asked focused on the physical and chemical properties of ether, in particular, the great effect temperature had over the relations of atmospheric air with the ether vapour. He had a head start. In 1808 the Manchester chemist John Dalton showed that the concentration of a vapour was determined by the temperature of air in which it was saturated. He published a table of comparative saturated vapour pressures of different liquids and, by chance, one of these was ether. Snow knew of Dalton's work so, using a eudiometer—a graduated glass tube, developed by Joseph Priestley and others in the thick of their researches into atmospheric air—he began to measure the amount of ether in air at different temperatures. Over and over he plunged the eudiometer containing air and ether over mercury into jars of water at various temperatures and carefully noted his results. He found that the temperature of the air in which the ether was vaporized was of crucial importance; as the temperature rose, so the amount of ether in the air increased. Dalton's rules held fast. His landlady, Mrs Williamson, was used to his home experiments—including the occasional explosion—but must have wondered at the powerful and unpleasant odour that drifted down from her lodger's rooms, permeating every room of the house.

Musing on the best way that ether could be inhaled by patients, Snow recalled an inhaler designed by Julius Jeffreys in 1842 for relieving chronic bronchitis by letting patients inhale warmed air. He visited Mr Daniel Ferguson, surgeon's instrument maker in Smithfield, an area notorious for its chaotic Monday morning market when the streets were filled with lowing oxen, crying sheep, and barking dogs as drovers brought hundreds of cattle to market. He briefed Ferguson on his plan of using Jeffreys' inhaler as a model and his desire to regulate the strength of the ether vapour through temperature. By 16 January Snow was ready to share his initial findings. He set out for the Westminster Medical Society.

Originally set up for students at the Windmill Street School of Medicine, the Westminster Medical Society was an established debating forum, attracting both physicians and surgeons. It was the first society Snow had joined soon after his arrival in London. On a dark January evening, members crowded into the elegant Georgian rooms in Savile Row, keen to share their experiences of the new 'ethereal agent'. Chairing the meeting was Henry Hancock, later to become President of the Royal College of Surgeons. Proceedings began with the exhibition of the uterus of a woman who had died during childbirth, though it was surely difficult to see the detail of inflammation in the flickering gaslight. The meeting swiftly moved on to the real subject of interest—ether.

Snow rose to address the physicians and surgeons, many of them senior men in the London hospitals who had been struggling to use ether. The problems they were experiencing—patients not 'going under', or waking up too soon—were occurring because of design faults in the inhalers, he began. Glass was a poor conductor of heat—many inhalers had been contrived out of glass vessels—and the ether inside such a container would cool rapidly and the vapour would condense out into liquid. Successful inhalation depended on enough vapour being inhaled. He spoke of his experiments to define the ratio between the temperature of the air and the amount of ether that would be taken up at that temperature, and explained the principle of the new instrument being made by Ferguson: made of metal, it would be placed in a basin of water which would allow the administrator to control the strength of the vapour. No inhaler currently in use in London had such a mechanism and this, said Snow, 'would account for some of the failures'. Discussion moved to some of the bad experiences. The physician William Merriman told of a case at St George's Hospital where, when the knife touched the patient, 'he bawled out and snatched his hand away'. At Westminster Hospital ether had brought 'delerium, convulsions, and almost asphyxia', despaired the surgeon Hale Thomson, and the similarity of ether's effects to drunkenness worried many.[42]

Snow returned with his new inhaler to the Society a week later, and in the shadowy light, demonstrated how the basin of water was 'brought to the desired temperature by mixing cold and warm water together', before ether was placed in the metal vessel with its interior spiral tin plate.[43] This mechanism spread the heat evenly and allowed the ether to vaporize and pass into the flexible tube and mouthpiece. Valves in the mouthpiece prevented the return of expired air. Snow had also paid great attention to the dimensions of the breathing tube to make sure it was not too wide, nor too narrow. Persuading patients to breathe a pungent vapour through tubes and valves was, he said, 'perfectly new'.[44] With his inhaler at the ready, he was keen to begin practice.

An accidental meeting was the catalyst. Snow later told his friend and biographer, Benjamin Ward Richardson, how he had bumped into a doctor he knew slightly who was 'bustling along' with a large ether apparatus under his arm. After exchanging greetings, the doctor said to Snow, 'Don't detain me, I am giving ether here and there and everywhere and am getting quite into an ether practice.' Reflecting on this as he walked on, Snow began to think that if it was possible for this doctor—with little scientific skill—to practise, then perhaps 'some scraps of the same thing may fall to a scientific unfortunate'.[45] St George's Hospital, sited on Hyde Park Corner, was one of the larger London hospitals and ether had been tried unsuccessfully on dental patients, many of whom were clamouring for the new pain relief. Snow, emboldened by his encounter, approached the hospital and was immediately appointed to the post. So impressive were his results that within days he was asked to give ether for surgery.

On 28 January in the round operating theatre, the floor covered with sawdust to soak up the blood, and watched by a group of surgeons and students, Snow put his new inhaler to work. Caesar Hawkins repaired an injury to the tibia of a young boy, Edward Cutler amputated a man's thigh, and Thomas Tatum removed a tumour from the shoulder of a Negro. There was no 'symptom of pain' and the patients did not remember anything of their operations although the Negro struggled a little to start with and Snow noticed that the veins in his forehead and arms became swollen during the inhalation. It was a sharp contrast to operations of earlier months where patients were bound, blindfolded, and held down as they endured the blade of the knife cutting through their skin or the

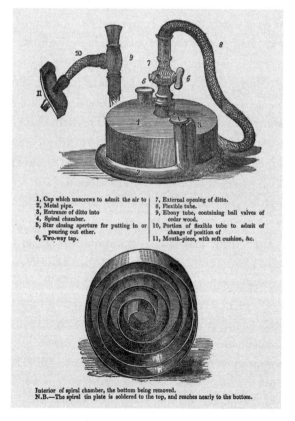

Figure 4 Snow's ether inhaler, modified to incorporate a two-way tap to control the supply of ether into the breathing tube.

insertion of a probe. After this experience Snow modified his inhaler to include a two-way cap of wide calibre to control the supply of the ether vapour into the breathing tube: 'The patient can begin by breathing unmedicated air, and have this gradually turned off as the etherised air is admitted in its place,' he explained.[46] By reducing the risk of initial coughing or spluttering, patients would become unconscious more quickly and the difficulties of excitement would be bypassed. The tap also allowed the administrator to maintain insensibility during the operation by giving a more diluted vapour.

Buoyed by his success, Snow approached Liston at University College Hospital. Enthusiastic about ether from the start, Liston was on the point of giving up because of the difficulty in effecting successful administrations. Snow began working with him and the problems were resolved. Liston was struck by Snow's skill and 'unaffected' nature but it was to be a short-lived partnership: Liston died unexpectedly in December 1847. Nevertheless Liston's support for Snow was hugely significant and within months Snow had almost exclusive command of London's ether practice.

In March 1847 some of the gloomy forebodings about ether seemed realized. Ann Parkinson, wife of a Grantham hairdresser, breathed ether whilst a tumour was removed from her thigh: she died thirty-six hours later, never having regained consciousness. An inquest was held to determine the cause of death. The jury decided that Mrs Parkinson died from the effects of ether. But they did not press charges against the surgeon as his intention—to save the patient the pain of surgery—was right and honourable. This decision set a precedent in Britain. Despite the many anaesthetic fatalities to occur during the nineteenth century, doctors were not held responsible for the vagaries of the anaesthetic's action, though they were beholden to administer the drugs as carefully as possible.

At the Essex and Colchester Hospital, the surgeon Roger Nunn read the reports of Ann Parkinson's death. It reminded him of one of his patients, Thomas Herbert, a 53 year old who had breathed ether during lithotomy a few weeks earlier, failed to recover, and died within hours of the operation. On reflection, Nunn decided that ether had depressed Herbert's nervous system beyond the point of recovery. By taking away the pain, said Nunn, ether removes 'the natural incentive to reparative action'.[47] That pain was purposeful and necessary was a long-held view. As seen in Chapter 1, ideas of pain started to shift in the late eighteenth century but many surgeons, like Nunn, continued to believe that it was an essential safety component of surgery. Should 'the great discovery of the age' be abandoned on account of these fatalities? asked the *Medical Times*. In Zurich and Hanover, laws had been passed to restrict the administration of ether to those with a medical degree in consequence of 'certain accidents'. One correspondent to *The Times* suggested that there should be a committee of enquiry on the matter: the question of ether was 'the largest' and 'the weightiest' to challenge the public and the profession. But ether was a watershed: once patients and doctors knew that it was possible to prevent the pain of operations it was impossible to pretend ether did not exist. As the French surgeon Joseph-Francois Malgaigne stated after amputating a workman's crushed limb under ether, 'I realised that on that day I was not writing surgical history but making it.'[48]

Snow continued to practice with ether—he developed a portable inhaler, much easier to carry round to the different homes and hospitals he visited, and promoted ether's benefits at every opportunity. On 12 May, taking some goldfish, birds, and guinea pigs with him, he went to lecture to military medical officers. In the luxurious surroundings of the United Service Club, Snow set up his glass jars of ether vapour and spoke of how difficult it would have been to anticipate ether: 'If any one had been asked last year whether it would be safe and practicable to induce such a state of insensibility as would prevent the most serious surgical operations being felt, and that without any ill consequences, he would, I think, undoubtedly have considered it an impossibility.' He showed how ether affected a thrush, guinea pig, and some goldfish, although the thrush unfortunately died as, distracted by his lecture notes, he forgot to take it out of the vapour soon enough. His advice was clear and direct: use an elastic tube in the inhaler so it can be kept out of the surgeon's way; start the patient inhaling air, and gradually build up the ether; otherwise the patient will start to cough. If you are the only medical man on board a small vessel, then get all your equipment ready, anaesthetize the patient, and then leave off the ether while you operate. He offered tips on preparing ether in tropical climes and emphasized its benefits on the battlefield:

> The pain endured by the bleeding sailor or soldier, wounded in fighting battles of his country, is deeply deplored by every feeling mind; and a discovery which can prevent so much of it, as depends on the operations necessary to save his life, must be hailed as a great blessing … for the pain of a surgical operation is greater than that of the wound itself … the approach of an operation is seen, and its cuts are necessarily deliberate; and though ever so expeditiously performed, it seems of immense duration to the patient.[49]

Neither Snow nor his audience knew that only a few years hence, on the battlefields of the Crimean War, some of the military officers would have to put his advice into practice.

A couple of months later Snow published *On the Inhalation of Ether in Surgical Operations*, which described the process of ether anaesthesia as five identifiable degrees which are still recognized in modern anaesthesia. Ether followed the same pathways in each body. It would initially affect the higher, more subtle brain functions and as its concentration in the blood increased, sensibility and movement would be suspended and the more important functions such as respiration would be steadily depressed. (In February Snow had decided that the state produced by ether was 'very different' from that of asphyxia.) The skill, of course, was to limit anaesthesia to the point where the core functions of the body were unimpaired. In Snow's view, although patients might respond differently to ether on the outside—girls might become giggly, men might become violent—on the inside of the body ether was systematic and predictable. Snow's work built on the new scientific idea of the body as a universal set of systems and organs which had emerged at the beginning of the nineteenth century. He was familiar with the French physician Xavier Bichat's 1800s experiments into states of life and death which showed how the process of death consisted of the gradual sequential elimination of functions, rather than the immediate cessation of life. Concussion, haemorrhage, or suffocation, or indeed breathing non-respirable gases, would first extinguish the higher functions of sensation, perception, and volition, before moving to the lower systems—the nervous system, circulation, and so on. Snow also drew on Flourens' 1824 experiments with pigeons which mapped the sequence of brain functions. (After the introduction of ether, Flourens had used these to show how ether followed a predictable pathway through the nervous system.) For Snow and a few other doctors like Francis Sibson in Nottingham, the new physiology provided the framework for understanding and administering ether.

By the summer of 1847 the initial furore surrounding ether had subsided. Like the Essex surgeon Roger Nunn, some doctors had abandoned ether, sometimes on physiological grounds, more often because they found it impossible to avoid the initial excitement. Successful ether administration demanded a mix of technical and people skills which not all doctors possessed. Sometimes, particularly when the ether was diluted, male patients struggled and female patients sobbed or screamed and tried to push away the inhaler. In such cases, advised Snow (who never failed with ether), the patient was guided by 'instinct rather than reason' and 'can often be quieted by language addressed to him, and will do as he is bid, although unconscious of where he is'. Nevertheless 'several eminent London surgeons' had given up with ether; they found the struggling impossible to accept, he added.[50] Across the border in Edinburgh, one physician was determined to find an alternative anaesthetic.

James Young Simpson was a strong advocate of ether from the start. He had ruffled feathers by giving it to mothers in labour: 'I am etherising all my obstetric cases, the ladies all demand it here. Nothing but good results here,' he wrote to his friend, London obstetrician Francis Ramsbotham.[51] Nevertheless, Simpson knew that ether's 'inconveniences and objections'—a pungent odour, tendency to irritate the throat and nasal passages, and initial excitement—were off-putting to patients and doctors alike. Thus he turned his attention to other volatile chemicals which might possess ether's 'advantages' without its 'disadvantages'. He broadcast his search widely; many chemists willingly supplied him with possible substitutes. In June 1847 he took on an assistant, Dr James Mathews Duncan, who became crucial to Simpson's enterprise. Behind the morning room in 52 Queen Street, Simpson's Edinburgh home, stood an oak cupboard containing bottles of the various chemicals Simpson had acquired during his search. Duncan was tasked to experiment with anything that had a smell or respirable vapour. Then, in the evening after dinner, Simpson, Duncan, and Dr Thomas Keith, a second assistant, would sit round the dining table inhaling various substances from tumblers or saucers. The routine was so well established that Simpson's friend and colleague, surgeon James Miller, popped into the house every morning to see how the previ-

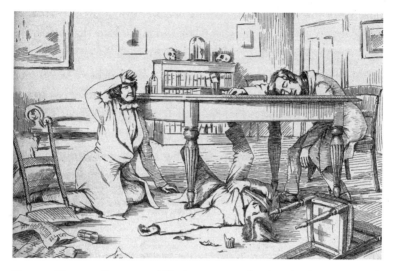

Figure 5 Simpson, Duncan, and Keith recovering after their first breathing of chloroform.

ous night's experiments had gone. On 4 November Duncan spent the morning sniffing various bottles. Then, as he later told his sister, he 'found himself awakening slowly and pleasantly from an unconscious sleep, which the timepiece showed must have lasted about a quarter of an hour'.[52] Simpson was told of Duncan's experience and agreed that the chemical should be tested that night. After dinner, Simpson, Duncan, and Keith charged their tumblers with the promising chemical which, they observed, had a delicious aroma. How bright-eyed, happy, and loquacious the doctors became, and how unusually intelligent the conversation, observed Simpson's wife Jessie, her niece Miss Petrie, and Simpson's brother-in-law. Then, all went quiet. Simpson, now prostrate on the floor, came round first: 'this is far stronger and better than ether'. Then he saw Duncan beneath a chair, quite unconscious and snoring loudly; Keith was lying on the floor with his feet and legs thrashing the table.

When calm resumed the doctors began inhaling again, then Miss Petrie had a turn: 'I'm an angel! I'm an angel! Oh, I'm an angel!', she cried as she fell asleep. Next morning Simpson ordered supplies of the chemical—chloroform—from Edinburgh chemists Duncan and Flockhart: it is said that they had to burn the midnight oil in order to meet Simpson's requirements. Within ten days Simpson had given chloroform to around fifty patients, though he had a near catastrophe with the first surgical patient. Miller had asked Simpson to give chloroform for a major operation but Simpson was unavoidably delayed; as the knife cut the skin the patient died. Chloroform would have been blamed for the death.

Like ether, chloroform was a known antispasmodic agent, listed in British pharmacopoeias since the late 1830s. Flourens had experimented with chloroform on animals but dismissed it as too lethal for patients. In October 1847 David Waldie, chemist to the Apothecaries Company in Liverpool, suggested to Simpson that chloroform had anaesthetic potential. He was to provide a sample but owing to various difficulties following the destruction of his laboratory by fire, failed to do so. Simpson never acknowledged Waldie's involvement, nor indeed Duncan's, claiming all glory for himself.

Simpson was zealous in promoting chloroform. On 10 November he announced his discovery to the Medical and Chirurgical Society of Edinburgh and on 15 November published a pamphlet, *On a new anaesthetic agent, more efficient than sulphuric ether.* Within days, 4,000 copies were sold and thousands more after. One copy was sent to Queen Victoria by her friend Harriet, Duchess of Sutherland. In London, Snow put chloroform to the test immediately he learnt of Simpson's discovery. He also breathed it himself until he felt very sick. It certainly had greater advantages for patients, but 'greater care was required in its use to avoid accident', warned Snow.[53] Worldwide, chloroform was delighting doctors and patients with its pleasant odour and ease of administration—there were no reports of failures.

Meanwhile Christmas arrived in Edinburgh: billboards promoted the *New Christmas Harlequinade* at the Theatre Royal, a theatrical extravaganza including *She Stoops to Conquer* and the Christmas comic pantomime *Children in the Wood*. Putting in an appearance for the first time was chloroform. During the pantomime the advertisement promised, the children would pass through several mysterious and magical scenes, including *Doctor Chloroform's Establishment* where 'the new anaesthetic agent and substitute for sulphuric ether' would aid operations without pain, arriving eventually in 'the grand and magnificent coral bowers of the silver fountains' where they would be reunited with 'the cruel Uncle and his unfortunate Wife in a state of poverty, upon which no agents, Anaesthetic or otherwise, have the least effect'.[54] That chloroform had become so notorious in six weeks or so is truly remarkable. But as 1848 gathered speed, the first chloroform fatality occurred and delight faded to fear.

Life had not been kind to 15-year-old Hannah Greener. Illegitimate and ill-treated when young, she had suffered great pain from her feet. In October 1847 she'd had one toenail removed under ether at Newcastle upon Tyne Infirmary: she felt no pain but complained of great heaviness to her head. On Friday 28 January she was to have a second toenail removed, this time under chloroform. The surgeon, Mr Meggison, and his assistant, Mr Lloyd, arrived at her home. Hannah was upset and apprehensive but the doctors were reassuring and seated her next to the fire. Whilst her stepfather held her foot, Meggison poured chloroform on a cloth and held it to her nose. 'I told her to draw her breath naturally … in about half a minute I observed muscles of the arm become rigid and her breathing a little quickened, but not sterterous,' Meggison later said.[55] When the knife began to cut her foot, Hannah jerked. Meggison thought

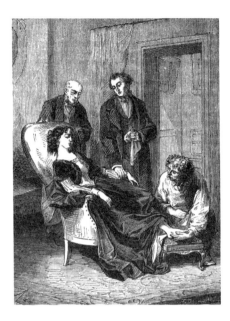

Figure 6 Hannah Greener, the first chloroform fatality who died on 28 January 1848.

she was not quite insensible but did not give any more chloroform. He opened her eyes and saw they were congested. He dashed water against her face and gave her brandy, a little of which was swallowed. Then he laid her on the floor, opened veins in her arm and neck, but to no avail. Less than three minutes after Hannah had breathed chloroform she was dead. That afternoon her body became the subject of a post-mortem inquiry.

Details of Hannah's death and subsequent inquest were reported in *The Times*; the medical press grappled to understand the cause of her sudden end. Sir John Fife, surgeon at Newcastle upon Tyne Royal Infirmary, assisted by Robert Mortimer Glover, lecturer at the medical school, performed the post-mortem. Glover had experimented with chloroform on animals in the early 1840s; his work had won him the Harveian Society gold medal. Intense congestion of the lungs was the most striking finding—it chimed with Glover's observation of congestion in the lungs of chloroformed mice after death. Fife told the jury, 'no human foresight, no human knowledge, no degree of science, could have forewarned any man against the use of chloroform in this case.' 'Hannah Greener died of congestion of the lung produced by [the direct effects of] chloroform,' concluded the jury. But the matter did not rest. Simpson challenged the verdict, arguing that the brandy and water given to Hannah had caused asphyxia, rather than the chloroform. Snow took a different view. After questioning Meggison on the details of Hannah's breathing, he decided death was caused by overdosage of chloroform. Hannah's movements could be matched to the different degrees of anaesthesia, he argued. Rigidity in her arm indicated she was in the third degree of anaesthesia, and though Meggison then removed the chloroform, its effects persisted for fifty seconds or so and brought her to the fifth degree, the point of no return. Chloroform had killed Hannah by poisoning her heart. The danger, said Snow, had arisen from Meggison's use of a cloth, rather than an inhaler.

Although numerous inhalers were developed during the first months of ether use, by 1848 most doctors had abandoned the technology, finding a sponge or cloth impregnated with chloroform and held over the patient's mouth and nose to be a far more effective method. A 'simple hanky', said Simpson, was all that was required: 'inhaling instruments frighten patients, whilst the handkerchief does not.'[56] Of course, the handkerchief would be made of silk for private patients. Snow championed a small group of practitioners who used inhalers on grounds of safety: the inhaler was a mechanism of quantifying dose and ensured anaesthesia remained within safe limits. Hannah's death provided a good opportunity to reiterate his message, and convince patients that chloroform was not to be unduly feared: 'I look on the result as only what was to be apprehended from the over-rapid action of chloroform when administered on a handkerchief ... and consider that danger may be avoided by adopting another method.'[57] Snow and Simpson's disagreements on the administration of chloroform and its mechanism of death defined the boundaries of a debate which outlasted both men. Until the twentieth century doctors disagreed as to whether chloroform killed through the respiration, or poisoned the heart.

Hannah Greener's death was vivid evidence of chloroform's propensity to kill without warning, whatever the medical disagreements about causes, and was followed by six further chloroform deaths during 1848: one in Britain, two in America, and three in France. One of the most interesting and startling aspects of the history of anaesthesia is that despite this early warning of chloroform's risks there was no return to ether in either Britain or most of Europe. It was 'almost impossible' for a doctor applying ether with 'ordinary intelligence and attention' to kill a patient, said Snow. Yet Snow, like other doctors, switched to chloroform and stuck to it: 'I use chloroform for the same reason that you use phosphorus matches instead of the tinder box. An occasional risk never stands in the way of ready applicability,' he explained.[58] In Snow's hands the risks of chloroform did seem to diminish: out of more than 4,500 anaesthetics he only suffered one chloroform fatality whereas best estimates suggest a fatality occurred in every 2,500 or so administrations. He did recommend ether to doctors not wishing to master the use of inhalers; even diluting the chloroform with alcohol could diminish the risks—but few took heed.

Over the course of the nineteenth century hundreds of chloroform fatalities were reported. The French surgeon J. E. Petrequin was one of the few European doctors who returned to ether in 1849:

Fatal accidents speedily occurred with us ... When I saw patients ... suddenly succumb to the action of chloroform, so that nothing could recall them to life and without the least warning of this catastrophe, I made up my mind as humanity dictated that I should. I abandoned the use of so dangerous an agent ... I had always found ether innocuous; it continued to give me good results without ever placing the patient's life in peril.

Petrequin's campaign to promote ether amongst French surgeons failed: 'ether was almost forgotten; there was an exaggerated admiration for chloroform. ... Nothing, in fact, could disillusion their minds.'[59] In America, Boston surgeons shared Petrequin's alarm of chloroform and returned to ether, though chloroform remained in use in the southern states. British medical use of chloroform reflected a national social tolerance of its risks, perhaps unmatched in other parts of the world. 'A good trial for manslaughter by a New England jury would bring British doctors to a quickened sense of responsibility,' noted an 1870 commentary in the *Boston Medical and Surgical Journal*. It encapsulated the different medico-legal climates enjoyed on each side of the Atlantic. Cases of medical malpractice suits had risen rapidly in America from the 1830s onwards. Once the dangers of chloroform versus ether were established, Boston doctors feared patients would sue them for choosing a more dangerous agent: the 'evidence to the jury would be unanimous that I might have employed ether, which is not fatal, and hence the responsibility of the fatality of chloroform ... [would rest] entirely on me,' explained ophthalmic surgeon Joy Jeffries in 1872.[60] British patients were far less likely to press charges against their doctor—none did for anaesthetic malpractice during the course of the nineteenth century. Patient tolerance of the risks of chloroform was driven by a strong fear of pain; an anxiety, it seemed, which overrode fear of death.

Ether and chloroform's powers to create oblivion to pain vindicated old promises that medical humanitarianism could improve life. Anaesthesia became synonymous with ideas of progress and the spread of civilization. But its risks, and how to mitigate them, were to occupy doctors for the remainder of the nineteenth century and beyond.

3

· · · ·

ANAESTHESIA IN ACTION

Patrick Brontë, father of Charlotte, Anne, Branwell, and Emily,
wrote to the *Leeds Mercury* in 1847:

> Every friend to humanity ought to cry 'all hail' to such a messenger of
> good tidings … Having read both sides of the question, and judging
> from the opinions of some of the most learned, able, and humane
> of the faculty, it appears to me to be evident, that as it regards the
> inhalation of the vapour of ether, a great, a useful, and important
> discovery has been made, and one that ought to be patronized by
> every friend to humanity.

He knew full well what the benefits of anaesthesia might be.

Whilst Morton was experimenting with ether in the summer of
1846, Patrick had travelled to Manchester to have a cataract removed
by William James Wilson, surgeon and founder of the Manchester Royal Eye Hospital. Patrick later documented his operation
in the margins of his medical bible—Graham's *Modern Domestic
Medicine*. 'Belladonna a virulent poison—was first applied, twice,
in order to expand the pupil—this occasioned very acute pains for
only about five seconds—The feeling under the operation—which
lasted fifteen minutes, was of a burning nature—but not intolerable.' To avoid post-operative infection, Patrick lay on his back in a

dark room for one month with bandages over his eyes, attended by a nurse; treatment included bleeding with leeches to prevent inflammation. His recovery was excellent. 'Through divine mercy, and the skill of the surgeon, as well as my Dr Ch's attention, and the assiduity of the nurse after a year of nearly total blindness—I was so far restored to sight, as to be able to read, and write, and find my way, without a guide.'[61] But it was a costly business, taking a quarter of his annual salary—even though Wilson had kindly reduced his fee to £10 from the usual £20–30.

Patrick was resigned to bearing the 'not intolerable' pain of his cataract removal. Painful surgery seemed one of the immutable facts of life before Morton's discovery. But his joyful response to ether underlines how strongly patients perceived anaesthesia to be the epitome of humanitarianism. For most patients, its advantages clearly outweighed its disadvantages though a minority found the pungency of ether unbearable, or were too fearful to try it. Some doctors grew convinced that anaesthesia should be a universal practice. John Snow's mantra—any patient fit for an operation was fit for anaesthesia, whatever their sex, age, or disease—was shared by James Simpson. But most employed anaesthesia selectively, judiciously limiting its use to those patients who seemed to present the least risk, or be in most need of pain relief.

It is hard for us to comprehend that for the first decades of anaesthesia not all patients received pain relief, nor did most doctors believe they should. That innovation brought new risks in its wake was widely acknowledged. Railways, steamboats, and stagecoaches had transformed travel and communication: they had also caused terrible accidents to life and limb, observed Simpson. Addressing critics, he pointed out that the new methods of travel had not been abandoned on account of accidents, but instead, accidents had become accepted as the unavoidable sting in the tail of progress. So should it be with the risks of anaesthesia, he proclaimed. His enthusiasm for distributing the new bounty of pain relief was unbounded. But many doctors found the risks to be alarming.

Under ether, states of life and death appeared to mingle. It was almost impossible for onlookers of an unconscious, pale, and insensible patient to know whether the patient was still alive: death appeared too close for comfort. The effects of ether on the body were appalling, noted Gideon Mantell, a Sussex surgeon and geologist, after watching operations at St Bartholomew's Hospital. Ether 'is not safe even when administered in a skilful manner', cautioned the *New York Journal of Medicine and Collateral Sciences*.[62] Prior to ether the state of deep insensibility and unconsciousness was associated with coma, extensive blood loss, suffocation, or drowning, conditions in which life hung on a thread.

Ether's effects on the body could be dramatic. The vapour seemed to exacerbate existing respiratory disease. In some instances patients' faces became purple and congested. Under ether, bleeding intensified and wounds healed slowly, bringing 'many obstacles to the skilful performance of an operation', lamented one London surgeon—we know now that it relaxes and dilates the blood vessels.[63] In some patients it appeared to cause convulsions, paralysis, and inflammation, and even changed the appearance of the blood. The experiments of James Pickford, a general practitioner in Brighton, suggested that ether caused black vitiated blood of the same kind found in putrid and malignant fevers. Ether was too dangerous, argued American army surgeon John B. Porter: 'the blood is poisoned, the nervous influence and muscular contractility is destroyed or diminished, and the wound is put in an unfavourable state for recovery ... hemorrhage is much more apt to occur.'[64]

Ether's power to create insensibility to pain was understood to derive from its intoxicating qualities thought to be similar to those of alcohol. Initially alcohol stimulated the body; its continued consumption depressed the body's systems until complete intoxication produced an insensible stupor. The story of the Irishman who had been so drunk as to lie on the ground whilst a pig chewed part of his face was well-known in medical circles; a wax model of his mutilated face was on display in the Park Street medical school in Dublin. Scotland too had its own example: the case of a man who complained to a magistrate that his testes had been cut off whilst he was in a drunken stupor at a wedding. Patients who inhaled enough ether would avoid the initial excitement and sink into unconsciousness and insensibility. But some, like the stout, masculine-looking female who breathed ether whilst the dentist James Robinson extracted a tooth, claimed that ether did not dull all sensation. Close questioning revealed that she had taken two glasses of gin 'to give her heart' for the operation: Robinson was reassured, as heavy drinkers or opium addicts were believed to be de-sensitized to ether's effects.

One of the most compelling concerns was the state of unconsciousness. What happened to the mind under ether? Time stood still for many patients: they awoke in the belief that the operation had not begun; only the evidence of an amputated stump or dressed wound convinced them otherwise. Even those who muttered or moaned throughout the operation experienced no sensations of pain. Vivid and hallucinatory dreams were common. Some were pleasant: 'an enjoyment too quickly passed away', noted one commentator. Others were disturbing and dragged the self into dark hinterlands: 'the dream is of drowning; a gushing in the ears, a choking and a sense of being lost, without pain or struggle or effort to save one's self,' recalled one patient.[65] The mind-altering effects of narcotics like opium were well established and addicts like the poet Samuel Taylor Coleridge knew full well the deep horrors of opium nightmares. Disturbing dreams were thus explained. But did the loss of consciousness have long-lasting effects?

During the late 1840s public concern about insanity was at a peak—in 1845 every county in Britain had been forced through legislation to create an asylum for the insane poor. Early psychiatrists like John Connolly pioneered new models and classifications of mental diseases and advocated moral therapy where the mad were treated like ill-behaved children, rather than physically restrained and punished. But there was little consensus as to whether madness originated from organic or environmental causes. It seemed possible that a short period of unconsciousness under ether could permanently damage the mind, or even change personality. (Simpson was swift to point out that anaesthesia was like sleep: no one suffered long-term damage from that.) Anaesthesia revealed only the truth, stressed the German surgeon Johann Langenbeck: 'ether will set the pious praying, the bully to draw his dagger and the loafer to carouse in the tavern. The dreamer may hear music, look at a pleasing landscape, sit at a well-laid table or cuddle a pretty maiden.'[66] Snow, in London, echoed his view: '*in vino veritas* was a proverb as applicable to Chloroform as to alcohol; and under no circumstances would "moral" women use "immoral" expressions,' he confidently affirmed.[67] Indeed anaesthesia could be a blessing for women. In hospitals students would crowd round to watch operations; women could now be put to sleep with just a nurse and doctor in attendance and unconsciousness would protect their female modesty from the spectacle. (Before operations on their vaginal area Snow always put women to sleep before their legs were raised and strapped.) Other doctors remained convinced that anaesthesia removed the subtle barrier between civilization and bestiality—between proper and improper behaviour.

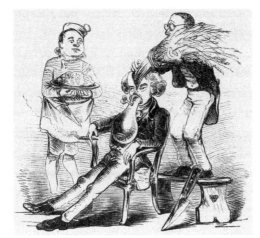

Figure 7 (*left*) Ether shown to be the cure-all for stupidity as it enables a head full of straw to be replaced by a brain painlessly.

Figure 8 (*below*) Ether shown to be the cure-all for ugliness as, without pain. A lady has one head removed and replaced by a prettier one.

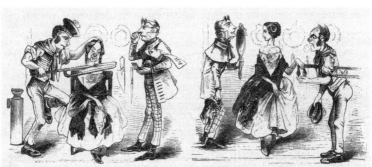

Ether could be intoxicating and exciting, releasing inhibitions and causing loquaciousness. 'Oh dear, I am falling,' cried Jane Evans who became hysterical whilst breathing ether at Liverpool Hospital before the removal of a cataract. The operation proceeded without pain although on recovery, Jane retained 'the sensation of falling': a glass of wine restored her to 'perfect consciousness'.[68] Some Victorian ladies, bound in the social straitjacket of morals and propriety, were unsettled by ether's power to unlock self-control. Charlotte Brontë, whose immediate thought on learning of ether was that she could have her front teeth 'extracted and rearranged', became alarmed by tales of its effects on her acquaintance, Catherine Swaine: '[I] would think twice before I consented to inhale; one would not like to make a fool of oneself,' she confided to her friend Ellen Nussey.[69] It was not so much the loss of patient self-control as the abnegation of consciousness that concerned some commentators.

Anaesthesia may create more problems than it solved, cautioned the Viennese professor of dentistry Moritz Heider. Imprudent and unconscientious dentists may be tempted to 'operate with still less care than they would otherwise', he warned, 'teeth might be broken or unnecessarily removed, the soft tissues might be injured'.[70] Some cartoons satirized such fears by depicting patients awaking to find the dentist had removed every tooth in their head. Other images suggested that by removing pain, ether brought a new world of possibilities in its wake. Not only could teeth be rearranged in the mouth, as Charlotte Brontë imagined, but painless surgery could transform appearances and intellectual powers.

It was not only patients who had to adjust to the new environment created by anaesthesia. Since antiquity, surgeons had looked to patients to assist them during certain operations by clenching muscles, or adopting a particular position: 'a surgeon must be well assisted by the patient or he cannot succeed,' wrote Robert Liston in his *Lectures on Surgery* (1846). Operations for fistulae, for example, were performed with the patient standing and bending over a table. If ether reduced patients to insensible motionless bodies then new strategies had to be sought. Beyond the practical there also loomed the moral implications of unconsciousness: 'with the doubtless laudable goal of operating without pain, they intoxicate their patients to the point of reducing them to what one could term the state of a cadaver which one cuts or carves with impunity and without any suffering,' chastised the French physiologist Francois Magendie.[71]

For most surgeons, the humanitarian benefits of removing pain sufficed to quell moral anxieties: history would judge harshly surgeons who advocated the benefits of painful operations, warned Simpson, whose ethical calculus prioritized the relief of pain.

One of the strongest fears was that ether would encourage unnecessary operations. A mania for operations has broken out in London, exclaimed the *Lancet*. Across the world the *Australian Medical Journal* cautioned against 'a FASHION ... the RAGE just now for ether' after operations under ether were performed in Sydney in June 1847.[72] Comparisons of operations performed pre- and post-ether in London and Boston suggest numbers of procedures more than doubled. But there is no evidence that this dramatic increase was sustained by unnecessary or experimental operations. Rather it is accounted for by patients with long-standing problems, who, perhaps, had previously refused operations for fear of pain. At St George's Hospital 13-year-old Thomas Hood had his thigh amputated under ether in February 1847 after suffering disease in his knee joint for many years. Francis Clayton, a countryman, had been troubled with loose cartilages in his knee joint for eleven years until they were removed in August 1847. Before anaesthesia patients would often procrastinate about operations and untreated minor injuries became sources of infection. The promise of pain relief persuaded reluctant patients to agree to surgery. In London's St Katharine's Docks in January 1847 a cask of sugar fell on the leg of a workman, causing a compound fracture. The patient refused to consent to an operation, said the surgeon, until he was promised it could be done without pain, using ether.

Debates on chloroform, which largely replaced ether as an anaesthetic from November 1847 onwards, centred on its physiological risks, especially the function of pain. Before ether, Edinburgh surgeon James Miller had noted the advantages of operating speedily on patients: 'The mere absence of protracted pain confers a most important advantage on the reparative powers of the system.'[73] Snow's argument was simple and compelling:

> A great part of the danger of an operation consists of the pain of it, which gives a shock to the system from which it is sometimes unable to recover ... Before the operation [anaesthesia] ... will supply the cordial of hope. During the operation it will prevent faintness which arises more from pain than loss of blood, which is seldom great.[74]

Yet old views, that pain was essential and diminished the risks of surgery, held ground. Pain was construed as a natural phenomenon that fulfilled a key function in nature's design. 'We had always understood that pain was given us as a blessing,' wrote one surgeon in a treatise on the rectum.[75] Doubt was cast on 'any process that the physicians set up to contravene the operations of those natural and physiological forces that the Divinity has ordained us to enjoy or to suffer', warned Charles Meigs, Professor of Obstetrics at the Jefferson Medical College, a lifelong opponent of anaesthesia. Surgical pain relief was 'a questionable attempt to abrogate one of the general conditions of man', argued Meigs.[76] Riding and railway travelling abrogate such general conditions, countered Simpson.

One strategy used by surgeons to diminish risk was to exclude patients with chronic diseases—heart conditions, respiratory disease, epilepsy, and so on. Another was to restrict anaesthesia to major operations, even though the smaller operations, such as toenail removal, were known to cause intense pain. (Hannah Greener had been having her toenail removed.) Chloroform should not be risked in 'trivial' operations, affirmed the *Lancet*. But seven fatalities in London in only eighteen months prompted the journal to strengthen its policy: 'Was the intensity or duration of the pain in an amputation of the leg sufficient to justify the fatal risk in such a subject? Or can it be said that insensibility was essential to the surgeon's proceeding?

Surely not,' expounded the journal after a further death at Guy's Hospital in 1854.[77] We do not know how many surgeons accepted the *Lancet's* views but the use of anaesthesia was certainly restricted, even for ex-prime ministers.

Favourite of Queen Victoria and stalwart of Parliament, Sir Robert Peel was riding in Hyde Park on 29 June 1850 when his horse began kicking and bucking. Peel was thrown over its head; the horse trampled on top of him. Passers-by rushed to help and Peel was taken home to Whitehall Gardens where the dining-room table served as a bed. Peel's collarbone, several ribs, and his leg were broken; the fragments of bone caused bleeding under the skin. Peel suffered 'excessive sensitiveness to pain', said his eminent doctors, Sir Benjamin Brodie, late President of the Royal College of Surgeons, and St George's Hospital surgeon Caesar Hawkins, and could not bear to be examined. Leeches were used to reduce the inflammation; his injuries were bandaged but this caused Peel excruciating pain. Over three days Peel gradually weakened and the effects of his injuries took their toll: no post-mortem was performed but it seems that pneumonia had set in and on 2 July Peel died. The nation mourned as if 'over a father', said Queen Victoria: on the day of his burial, factories stopped, shops shut, and flags were lowered to half mast.[78] Reflecting on the incident many years later, Brodie's biographer mused that if Peel had been put under chloroform 'it might have been easy to have put the broken bone in place, or removed it, and if necessary secured the wounded vein', but, he noted, 'all this was out of the question at the time'.[79] Brodie and Hawkins were both familiar with chloroform at the time of Peel's death. Either they deemed the risks too great to offer it to Peel, or he refused it. It is a sad story.

One of the problems of restricting anaesthesia to certain groups of patients was the difficulty of accounting for individual sensibility.

Like Peel, some patients were excessively sensitive to pain whereas others bore pain stoically and with fortitude. Doctors explained such differences through the classical view of the body in which each patient was understood to respond differently to the stress and pain of an operation. In May 1851, without the benefit of anaesthesia, John Hoare, a porter, was placed on his knees and elbows at Guy's Hospital whilst the surgeon, Hilton, tried to locate a fistula in his rectum, first with a probe, then a speculum, but with no success: the operation was abandoned. Hoare was put to bed having 'borne the operation heroically and only complained of smarting in the parts'. Other patients suffered more intensely as the sorry tale of William Guscott shows. Admitted to King's College Hospital for lithotomy in 1850, Guscott suffered great pain whilst the surgeon, William Fergusson, passed a small sound into his bladder and detected a stone—chloroform was not given. The same evening, depressed by the prospect of a further operation, Guscott tried to hang himself. He was resuscitated but died after two days. Surgeons knew only too well that a patient's outlook strongly determined the outcome of an operation. Expressions like 'frightened to death ... are not always mere figures of speech', wrote the physician C. J. B. Williams.[80] Numerous instances of sudden death during surgery before anaesthesia had no cause other than fear or pain, noted Snow in 1858.

Sensibility was also thought to be differentiated by sex, age, and class. Women had long been thought to be more sensitive to internal and external sensations and by the nineteenth century doctors agreed that female physiology underpinned every characteristic—mind, emotions, behaviour, health, and strength—of a woman. Women's destiny as the nation's daughters, wives, and mothers was determined by biology. Separating life into private and public spheres created environments honed to enhance the natural characteristics of males and females, asserted physician Michael Ryan.

Subordination of women to men was expected at a physical and intellectual level. It was also reinforced by law which ruled that married women relinquished ownership of property or assets to their husbands. Equally, arguments about male physiology—its strength and rationality—reinforced notions of male supreme authority and their ability to hold positions in public life. It was a complex dichotomy because at the same time that women were characterized as physically and intellectually subordinate to men, they were also deemed to have greater moral and physical sensibilities. Women were the guardian angels of social morality. Such convictions infused the literature of the day. 'You have deep responsibilities, you have urgent claims; a nation's moral wealth is in your keeping,' stated Mrs Sarah Stickney Ellis in 1839.[81] Ellis wrote widely on the duties of women, as daughters, wives, and mothers, to shape the moral character of the nation by living a selfless and exemplary life. The 'highest duty' of women was to 'suffer and be still', she frequently reminded readers.[82] Women 'shed on domestic society that benign humanising influence, which her moral constitution, when purified and elevated by Christian religion, is so eminently fitted to exercise', noted surgeon and obstetrician J. Roberton in 1851.[83] Such views severely limited the access of middle-class women to education, work, and financial independence, even though thousands of their working-class counterparts laboured for long hours and looked after a family. What middle-class women did gain though was better access to anaesthesia.

A woman, said Oliver Wendell Holmes, who advised Morton on the naming of anaesthesia, is 'much more fertile in capacities of suffering than a man. She has so many varieties of headaches!'[84] 'In many individuals of the softer sex there is so great a degree of physical as well as mental sensibility, that they cannot bear a great amount or long continuance of pain. The patient either sinks at once under her sufferings, or a lingering disease is induced,' asserted Edward Warren, brother of John Collins Warren, the first surgeon to operate with Morton.[85] Though united in the desirability of pain relief for women, doctors feared that the susceptibility of the female system increased its risks: 'In females and children ... the action of chloroform is quicker, more complete, and therefore more dangerous,' wrote Morton, perhaps reflecting his allegiance to ether.[86] And female propensity to hysterics put them on a par with 'lively excitable animals', said one British surgeon, writing in the *American Journal of Medical Sciences*.[87] Snow was equable in his approach, persisting with inhalation until the effects of the anaesthetic overrode the hysteria: 'I do not consider that the hysterical diathesis forms any objection to the use of chloroform in operations, as the patients would generally be quite as liable to suffer an attack of hysteria from the pain, if chloroform were not used.'[88] However, when a young married lady suffered a 'somewhat violent paroxysm of hysteria' whilst inhaling chloroform, the surgeon forbade Snow to continue. As the hysteria had not abated after half an hour, Snow began again, this time rendering the patient insensible. Most surgeons avoided operating on women during menstruation for fear of exacerbating their hysterical tendencies, supposedly worse at this time. Snow was nonchalant: 'I have seen no ill-effects from it,' he remarked.

Male sensibility was a different matter. Stoicism in the face of pain was a manly quality. 'A strong, full-blooded man is pretty sure to resist [the anaesthetic process],' asserted the Boston Society for Medical Improvement in 1861.[89] The most common example of manly strength was resilience on the battlefield: 'heroic manly fortitude, heightened by the exhilaration of a good fight, makes soldiers almost insensitive to the pain of almost any operation,' boasted John B. Porter, surgical chief of the American army.[90] Indeed strong, muscular patients were the most difficult to anaesthetise on account of their struggling. The most violent struggling under chloroform Snow recorded occurred in a celebrated harlequin working in London's theatres.

Race also determined the use of anaesthesia. Medical arguments surrounding patient selection hinged on the idea that coloured races had much less sensitivity to pain. 'The savage does not feel pain as we do,' noted American physician Silas Weir Mitchell.[91] Childbirth was the most popular example of differentiated racial sensibility. 'Woman in a savage state ... enjoys a kind of natural anaesthesia during labour,' commented Simpson: mothers in civilized societies suffered intensely, though again sensibility was differentiated by class.[92] Working-class mothers in Manchester gave birth in a state of 'extreme apathy', remarked the surgeon Charles Clay in 1842.[93] Intensified sensibility seemed a curious and worrying backlash of civilization. The spread of civilization creates 'a delicacy of feeling, that disposes alike to more acute pain, as to more exquisite pleasure', surgeon Thomas Trotter had cautioned in his *Review of the Nervous Temperament* (1808). James Marion Sims developed new techniques for repairing vesicovaginal fistulas by experimenting on three Negro women in Alabama, performing around thirty operations on each between 1845 and 1849—all without anaesthesia. Such fistulas were often caused by difficult labours and led to persistent incontinence. The benefits of Sims's refined techniques were indubitable and benefited generations of women. Yet his attitudes to sensibility were rooted in his times: he had chosen Negro women, he explained, not because they were slaves and bound to comply, but for their high pain thresholds: white women were too sensitive to endure such an experience.

Like women, the young and the old were thought to be especially vulnerable to suffering. Children responded well to ether and chloroform and showed less initial excitement and struggling. Surgeons in Boston and London were more likely to give anaesthesia to children than to adults undergoing the same operation. On a practical level, anaesthesia enabled surgeons to control young patients as never before and allowed the performance of particularly painful procedures such as lithotrity—crushing bladder stones and leaving fragments to dispel. Prior to ether, lithotrity was deemed unsuitable for children. Snow advocated anaesthesia for the very youngest of infants, even those who were only days old. But Henry J. Bigelow, surgeon at Massachussetts General Hospital, took a different view, arguing that because very young children neither anticipated nor remembered pain, anaesthesia was not required.

The easiest way, of course, to avoid anaesthetic risk and still perform operations without pain was to use an alternative method. In 1847 the Brighton Infirmary surgeon James Arnott pioneered congelation—the use of cold. Only a simple apparatus was required, he said: a small pig's bladder, some pounded ice, and a little salt were used to numb the skin to a temperature below freezing point which rendered it insensible to the knife. Arnott campaigned long and hard against anaesthesia's dangers, publishing pamphlets and demonstrating his method in Paris and London. Congelation was not just safe, he stressed, but also cheap: 'On one occasion, in employing congelation in phlebitis, I borrowed for the purpose the net which confined the hair of the attendant nurse; and the principal ingredient cost as little as the instrument which contained it, for, there being a snowstorm at the time, it was gathered from the door-step.' Some surgeons used congelation occasionally, though 'the skin does not cut as crisp as natural when frozen, but like tough soap, requiring a little modification in the handling of the scalpel', warned James Paget, surgeon at St Bartholomew's Hospital.[94] But cold could not compete with the quality of insensibility produced by ether and chloroform.

Evidence suggested that despite its risks, anaesthesia improved surgical outcomes, though the hazards of infection and blood loss continued. Simpson gathered statistics to show that under ether, the mortality rate in British hospitals for amputations of the thigh, leg, and arm had dropped from twenty-nine to twenty-three deaths per hundred cases. In amputation at the thigh—the most dangerous amputation—the death rate had fallen from 1 in 2 patients to 1 in 4. Snow gave Simpson his results from St George's Hospital, which showed a mortality rate of 10 per cent far below the average of 20 per cent for all hospitals. It could be that the availability of pain relief encouraged some patients to submit to an operation at an earlier stage of disease that they might otherwise have done, thereby altering previous patterns. But figures could not dispel medical fears. In London hospitals, anaesthesia remained a selective practice until the 1860s. For patients who could afford to pay for medical care, matters were slightly different.

Private patients were treated in their homes or the doctor's rooms. Those living in the country would, like Patrick Brontë, travel to the nearest city to see a doctor. If a programme of treatment or an operation was required, they would take lodgings or stay in a hotel. Thousands of operations on the middle classes, attended by family or friends, were performed in these settings. Hospitals remained the preserve of the poor and working classes for much of the nineteenth century. Surgeons and physicians appointed to hospital posts would receive small payments but the bulk of their income derived from private practice. In hospitals, institutional authority and surgical autocracy was a powerful combination. If anaesthesia was deemed too risky it would be withheld. Beyond hospital walls, succeeding in private practice depended much on pleasing patients. Doctors had no illusions about patient loyalty: most patients chose anaesthesia rather than suffer pain. In 1854 Snow gave chloroform to an elderly gentlemen whilst several teeth were extracted. The patient had suspected heart disease: anaesthesia was too risky, advised his usual doctor, but sent him for a second opinion which reiterated the dangers. Despite these two warnings, the patient 'resolved to have chloroform' if Snow thought it right to give it to him, though he avoided telling his family his plans in advance of the operation which had no unpleasant side effects. Other patients were not so lucky. A lady about to have a breast amputated demanded chloroform but collapsed: 'her face was of a deadly pallid and livid colour, and her lips, lobes of the ears and fingernails, of a deep purple hue.' She had to be resuscitated, reported Charles Bleeck to the *Lancet* in 1850.[95] Administering anaesthesia remained incidental to the working lives of most doctors. But in London, Snow carved out a new medical role—the anaesthetist.

Snow features large in the history of anaesthesia, partly for his establishment of its scientific principles and leadership of London practice, partly for the wonderful evidence we have of his daily anaesthetic work. The pages of his surviving casebooks, dating from 1848 to 1858, record almost 4,500 anaesthetic administrations on patients of all ages, nationalities, and personalities. He worked with over 100 surgeons and around 70 dentists, giving anaesthetics at all the major London hospitals and numerous hotels, lodgings, and dental practices. Some patients travelled long distances from the Lake District, Bolton, Leeds, Chester, and the Isle of Wight. Others hailed from far-flung places: America, France, China, and Australia. One 5-year-old girl travelled from Bombay. Snow gave her chloroform whilst the surgeon, William Fergusson,

> scooped out some polypus growth from the right nostril and also an oval, softened body rather bigger than a horse bean, said to be a young orange that the child had pushed up the nostril in India. The case had given rise to a good deal of difference of opinion amongst medical men in India and Malta.[96]

Some patients were more memorable than others: one was ' a believer in table-moving, and believes she can make a saucer move towards her on the table, by her will, without touching it', Snow noted wryly.

Successful anaesthesia required exemplary patient management and the casebooks make clear the extent to which Snow was recog nized as an expert within, and beyond London. Dr Ferguson tried to dissuade his patient, Mrs Hawes, from inhaling chloroform whilst she had two teeth extracted. He was concerned because she suffered from epilepsy and was also breastfeeding her baby. He decided to send her to Snow: 'she might have it [chloroform] if I saw no objection,' noted Snow. Mrs Hawes inhaled easily and recovered well, saying the flavour and effects of chloroform were 'very pleasant'.[97] Much is made of Snow's dour Yorkshire personality but his observation of character was acute and his skill in managing patients from all walks of life is evident. In April 1850 he attended the first Marquess of Anglesey who was suffering intense pain in his stump. Injured whilst serving as second in command to Wellington, at Waterloo, the Marquess had an above-knee amputation after the battle in 1815. His bravery during the amputation was well known: he remained still, his pulse rate unchanged, and only commented on the bluntness of the surgeon's saw. Aged 82 years in 1850, he still suffered acute attacks of pain in the stump. Snow began by applying chloroform to the site but the pain remained so the Marquess inhaled it. It exhilarated and enlivened him, said Snow: the inhalation was repeated several times until the pain subsided. Whilst Snow was attending to the stump, the Marquess received notice of the death of an artillery man on board a navy ship in Mauritius a few months earlier. The man had been given chloroform on a handkerchief before his finger was removed but then turned pale and his breathing and pulse stopped—he could not be revived. Some patients may have been deterred from inhaling, said Snow: the Marquess was indomitable. A few weeks later Snow attended him again when, under the influence of chloroform, the Marquess made a speech as if addressing a meeting or a dinner party.

Often patients needed reassurance and sympathy, particularly fearful lady patients like Mrs Dickinson, who suffered palpitations and was greatly apprehensive of chloroform: 'the pallor consequent on fear disappeared' as the anaesthetic took effect, observed Snow.[98] Sometimes surgical fears had to be allayed: 'Mr Dixon [the surgeon] had entertained some objection to the use of chloroform in this case, but its effects were very satisfactory,' Snow noted in 1852.[99] At other times surgical autocracy interfered with good anaesthesia; for example, Snow recorded in May 1854:

> Mr S. performed the operation in this case without waiting till I told him. I saw him doing something and told him the patient was not insensible. He said 'I know better. I am doing the operation and he does not move'. The patient, who was not even quite unconscious, was looking up in my face at the time. After the operation I went up to Mr Salmon and told him in an undertone that I thought the patient had been conscious of the operation. I then went back to the patient and asked him how he was. He said 'Very Bad'. ... He immediately fell into a state of syncope, accompanied with ... convulsions during which he slid partly out of bed, but being lifted in again, and his face being well-slapped by Mr Salmon with the corner of a towel dipped in water. The patient recovered in a minute or two. ... He told us that he felt the operation.

Like other doctors, Snow experimented widely with ether and chloroform in a range of diseases: asthma, epilepsy, rabies, tetanus, and epidemic fevers like cholera. Snow, of course, is remembered as much for his work on cholera as on anaesthesia. He witnessed the devastation wrought by the 1831–2 cholera epidemic when he was sent to care for the miners in Killingworth colliery. Cholera returned with a vengeance in 1848—less than twelve months after the introduction of chloroform—and this epidemic claimed over 53,000 victims in England and Wales. Feared beyond all other infectious diseases, cholera began with severe diarrhoea, colourless and odourless with the appearance of 'rice water', often accompanied by vomiting and severe abdominal pain. The patient then moved to the 'blue stage', becoming cold with clammy skin and sunken, dull eyes. Death was speedy and violent. Once the illness started, most victims survived no more than twenty-four hours, and often died within twelve hours of the first symptoms, their corpses bearing the ghostly death visage of cholera. Such was the urgency to rid houses and streets of cholera corpses that tales abounded of victims being buried alive in the overflowing graveyards. Nor was this peculiar to Britain. The Belgian artist Antoine Wiertz, known for his morbid fascination with death, painted a coffin with a raised lid and a hand creeping round its edge in protest at the precipitate burial of the 'not quite dead' during the 1854 cholera epidemic in Brussels.

During the 1848 outbreak of cholera in London, Snow gathered together evidence from family and associates to analyse the spread of the epidemic, eventually surmising that contaminated water was the main vehicle of transmission. In 1849 he published his theory and guidelines on stopping the spread of the disease. Drinking water was contaminated by the cholera evacuations of the sick seeping into wells or entering rivers from which drinking water was collected, he explained. Great attention should be paid to cleanliness in the sickroom, particularly in the handling of chamber pots and soiled bed linen; simple measures like boiling and filtering drinking water were highly effective, he advised. His theory won him few allies: reviews of his pamphlet were lukewarm; it was 'a modest contribution to medical literature on cholera', acknowledged the *London Medical Gazette*. Snow did not let the matter rest and continued to analyse new outbreaks, showing how cholera was spread through contaminated water. Only in 1854 did he obtain definitive proof of his theory through an outbreak of cholera in Broad Street where he traced the source of contaminated water to the local pump, and his investigation of the water sources of two of London's water companies showed again that cholera was spread through contaminated water supplies. This time he won some support and in 1855 gave evidence to a Parliamentary Select Committee. But the cause and spread of epidemic disease remained highly contested for many years although clean water was increasingly provided. In 1883 Snow's work was finally confirmed by Robert Koch's identification of the bacillus *Vibrio cholerae* in 1883, which showed how the bacillus lived in the intestine and spread primarily through contaminated water. Snow combined both his interests when he used chloroform to relieve the symptoms of cholera victims.

Chloroform could not cure cholera but it could buy rest from the exhausting progression of the disease. In 1849 Snow gave it to Mrs McAllister who was suffering severe cramps and 'almost constant vomiting'. Inhaling chloroform allowed her to fall into a natural sleep—surprisingly, she recovered.[100] Snow also used chloroform on Mr Webb, living in one of Soho's filthy, cramped dwellings:

> vomiting and retching constantly, complaining of severe cramps and of pain … the state of unconsciousness merged into a natural sleep … a quarter of an hour afterwards he opened his eyes and, on being questioned, said that he was easier. He immediately fell asleep again, and slept till about two hours … in the morning was better.[101]

But a few days later he died of suppression of urine. The use of chloroform in such cases prompted few criticisms. Against the fatal powers of cholera, the risks of anaesthesia seemed by far the lesser of two evils.

Doctors differed sharply on the conundrum of anaesthetic risk in surgery and dentistry until at least the 1860s, though patient support for pain relief was strong from the beginning. The most heated debates took place in relation to childbirth anaesthesia. Here, as we will see, patient persistence won through.

4

. . . .

WOMEN, SEX,
AND SUFFERING

'I never was better or got through a confinement so comfortably, I feel proud to be the pioneer to less suffering for poor, weak womankind,' enthused Fanny Longfellow, wife of poet Henry Wadsworth Longfellow, who inhaled ether during the birth of her daughter Fanny, on 7 April 1847. Fanny was the first mother to use ether in childbirth in the USA—she had struggled to find a physician willing to administer it. Eventually Nathan Keep, Dean of Dentistry at Harvard University, agreed to help. Keep had used ether successfully in dental surgery and Henry Longfellow visited him to discuss its potential use in childbirth. The birth—Fanny's third confinement—went well. Her 'sufferings of the last moments were greatly mitigated' by ether and 'to the great joy of all', recorded Henry Longfellow in his journal, their first daughter was born at Craigie House, overlooking the Charles River in Cambridge, Massachusetts. 'I am very sorry you all thought me so rash and naughty in trying the ether,' Fanny later apologized to her family. 'Henry's faith gave me courage and I had heard such a thing had succeeded abroad, where the surgeons extend this great blessing much more boldly and universally than our timid doctors,' she explained. Her example was swiftly followed by two other ladies. Ether is 'the greatest blessing of this age, and I am glad to have lived at the time of its coming and in the country which gives it to the world', but how sad that 'such a gift of God' had been accompanied by squabbles over the priority of discovery, she continued. 'One would like to have the bringer of such a blessing represented by some grand, lofty figure like Christ, the divine suppressor of spiritual suffering as this of physical.'[102]

Women throughout the Western world would have empathized with Fanny's desire to relieve the pain of childbirth. Without reliable contraception, pregnancy was a familiar state to most married women who had to face the risks and suffering of childbirth on a regular basis. The statistics of the period make grim reading. The Registrar-General William Farr estimated that between 1847 and 1876 maternal mortality was just under 1 death in every 200 live births and it was to increase over the rest of the century. Infection introduced into the uterus by midwife or doctor during a delivery frequently caused puerperal fever. In the late 1840s Ignaz Semmelweis, physician at the Vienna General Hospital, discovered that handwashing with chlorinated water dramatically reduced deaths from this cause. Nevertheless, during the 1850s and 1860s puerperal fever caused between 33 and 38 per cent of maternal deaths in England and Wales; by the 1890s, it accounted for 50 per cent of maternal deaths. Twenty-six-year-old Margaret Gladstone talked to her husband, the scientist John Gladstone, about the risks of dying in childbirth: she contracted puerperal fever and died four weeks after the birth of their first child in 1870. Miscarriages could also be fatal. Henry Longfellow's first wife, Mary Potter, had died from a miscarriage in 1835. Even without the ultimate risk of death there was, of course, the pain and suffering of labour.

On many levels the pain of childbirth was understood to be natural and necessary. In the Christian tradition, suffering during labour provided a permanent reminder of Eve's original sin in the Garden of Eden and opponents of anaesthesia were swift to draw on the Biblical admonition that 'in sorrow shalt thou bring forth children'. Labour pains were understood to be natural phenomena and perform a necessary physiological function during birth: 'the reasons … actuating the physician to allow the inhalation of chloroform … must be exceedingly strong, or he will violate the law of non-interference with nature, founded on the experience of so many physicians of celebrity during a succession of years,' advised physician Samuel Merriman.[103] For this reason, many doctors vociferously opposed any efforts to subdue pain.

Across the Atlantic doctors united to protest against the dangers of anaesthesia in childbirth. Charles Meigs, Professor of Obstetrics at Jefferson Medical College in Philadelphia, objected passionately to medical interference in a natural process. So did London obstetrician William Tyler Smith: 'Women will derive truer comfort and a greater measure of safety and freedom from unnecessary suffering from physiology, than from wild therapeutics, which in her hour of trial only offer a choice betwixt poison and pain.' Ether's tendency to excite patients, especially when given in small doses, prompted concerns that it could create sexual excitement in labour. Tyler Smith believed the process of labour was on a par to sexual intercourse: it was only the pain of labour that kept a woman's feelings in check. If ether removed the pain then women would feel 'the sensations of coitus' rather than 'the pangs of travail'.[104] It was impossible to overstate the moral dangers arising from such a situation, he expostulated. Even ether's supporters struggled to rationalize its effects. Edward Murphy, Professor of Midwifery at University College London and colleague of Snow, found ether facilitated difficult births wonderfully—ones requiring forceps or other interventions—yet he was concerned that women appeared drunk and out of control.

But like Fanny, mothers-to-be were enthusiastic from the beginning. Fanny's entrancement with ether was shared by Scottish physician James Simpson. Only weeks after news of the Yankee dodge with ether reached Britain, Simpson gave it to a mother during a difficult birth: the labour was complicated by the mother's contracted pelvis. Ether did not save the baby but it did create 'gratitude and wonderment' in the patient. 'I can think of naught else,' wrote Simpson to his brother, claiming that the excitement of the event eclipsed even his new appointment as Queen Victoria's obstetrician in Scotland.[105] Simpson was the most vocal advocate for childbirth anaesthesia, defending its use on grounds of morality. Normal births caused women 'abundantly severe' suffering that matched the intensity of surgical pain. Doctors had accepted this phenomenon because there was no alternative. But now, Simpson argued, there was an alternative. Anaesthesia gave doctors 'the proud power of being able to cancel and remove pangs and torture that would otherwise be inevitable'. It would be immoral not to take the advantages it offered: 'I most conscientiously believe that the proud mission of the physician is distinctly twofold—namely to alleviate human suffering as well as preserve human life,' he affirmed.[106]

But some doctors continued to claim value in pain. To abolish pain was 'a dangerous folly', said the London obstetrician William Gull, and George Gream, obstetrician at Queen Charlotte's Lying-In hospital, drew ammunition from the views of eighteenth-century surgeon Thomas Denman, known for being the first licentiate in midwifery of the Royal College of Physicians and who wrote in the 1790s:

In everything which relates to the act of parturition, nature ... is fully competent to accomplish her own purpose ... all women should believe, and find comfort in the reflection, that they are at these times under the peculiar care of Providence, and that their safety in childbirth is ensured by more numerous and powerful resources than under any other circumstances.

To use chloroform was 'indiscriminate, unjustifiable, and wanton', ruled Gream.[107] But times had changed and so had patients, particularly in matters of pain.

Husbands will 'scarcely permit the sufferings of their wives to be perpetuated, merely in order that the tranquillity of this or that medical dogma be not rudely disturbed', Edinburgh physician James Moffat reminded his peers. Women themselves will 'rebel against enduring the usual tortures and miseries of childbirth'.

> I more than doubt if any physician is really justified, on any grounds, medical or moral, in deliberately desiring and asking his patients to shriek and writhe on in their agonies for a few months, or a few years longer, in order that, by doing so, they may ... pander to his professional predjudices.

Time, said Moffat, would prove the 'barbarity of leaving patients to painful suffering'.[108] Simpson tried to quell discontent by producing statistics which showed the benefits of anaesthesia, particularly in difficult births requiring forceps. He also anticipated that strong opposition may come from religious camps and prepared his armour. In the pamphlet, *Answer to the Religious Objections advanced against the employment of Anaesthetic Agents in Midwifery and Surgery*, Simpson argued that the meaning of the original Hebrew text—'in sorrow shalt thou bring forth children'—had been misrepresented. The word 'sorrow', he claimed, should be translated as labour, toil, or physical exertion. Chloroform relieved the real pain not referred to in the text, the labour or exertion of childbirth remained unhampered, and he insisted that employment of anaesthesia was in 'strict consonance' with the spirit of Christian dispensation. We do not know whether Simpson would have won the argument on religious grounds: the battle never took place. Only a few lone voices drew on Christian philosophies to protest: 'Chloroform is a decoy of Satan, apparently offering itself to bless women; but in the end it will harden society and rob God of the deep earnest cries which arise in time of trouble for help,' expostulated one clergyman in a letter to Simpson.[109]

Physicians like Simpson and Moffat were in tune with the times. Public support of childbirth anaesthesia was strong and, as Moffat had predicted, was driven as much by husbands as by wives. 'What an awful affair a confinement is!', noted Charles Darwin after the birth of his first child in 1839: the event 'knocked me up, almost as much as it did Emma herself'. Husbands as much as their wives seem to have been in favour of relieving the pain of childbirth. It may be that our examples come from enlightened thinkers: men like Charles Dickens, Charles Darwin, Robert Hooker, and, of course, Prince Albert. They were perhaps unusual for their time. Nevertheless their stories paint pictures of supportive husbands willing to challenge medical conservatism on the use of anaesthesia in childbirth to save their wives' suffering. For Charles Darwin unnecessary suffering flew against all civilized impulses. When a medical student in Edinburgh in 1826, Darwin had witnessed two operations without anaesthesia and fled before their completion. The agony and distress of the patients 'haunted me for many a long year', he noted and shortly afterwards abandoned his studies.[110] When later pondering on his experience, Darwin wondered how any naturally sympathetic individual could tolerate imposing suffering on another being. Emma, Darwin's wife, conceived their seventh child around the time Simpson announced his discovery of chloroform. Spurred on by his intense sensitivity to physical pain Darwin tried it himself and sought advice on its use in childbirth from Francis

Boott, one of the first to receive the news of ether from Boston. By May he affirmed to his friend Joseph Hooker that his and Emma's next child would be brought into the world 'under the influence of Chloriform'. Two days after the birth of Francis Darwin on 16 August 1848, Darwin wrote to Boott: 'with my true thanks for all your sympathy and assistance about Chloriform'. Darwin became chloroform's devotee. In 1850 Emma's labour came on unexpectedly: Darwin could not withstand her entreaties for chloroform so he soaked a pad with the chemical and held it over Emma's nose. It was exactly the situation that would have alarmed Snow. Darwin kept Emma unconscious for one and a half hours: there could have been fatal consequences but Darwin was untroubled. He wrote to his old Cambridge professor of botany, John Henslow, after the birth of his son, Leonard, on 15 January 1850.

> I was so bold during my wifes confinement which are always rapid, as to administer Chloroform, before the D$\underline{r}$ came & I kept her in a state of insensibility of 1 & ½ hours & she knew nothing from first pain till she heard that the child was born.—It is the grandest & most blessed of discoveries.

Darwin's enrapture remained: 'Did you administer the Chloroform?', he asked Hooker after the birth of his daughter in 1854, adding, 'I was perfectly convinced that the Chloroform was very composing to oneself as well as to the patient.'[111] Hooker had indeed followed Darwin's example.

Charles Dickens was equally adamant that his wife, Kate, should be saved the pain of childbirth. She had a history of difficult labours and miscarriages. When she fell pregnant in 1848 Dickens planned ahead and during a visit to Edinburgh, perhaps through consulting Simpson, made himself 'thoroughly acquainted with the *facts* of chloroform'. He promised Kate that she should have it. When labour commenced, Dickens insisted that the chloroform administrator from St Bartholomew's hospital attended the birth. He later wrote to his friend, actor William Macready, after the birth of his eighth child, Henry Fielding Dickens, on 16 January 1849:

> The doctors were dead against it but I stood my ground, and (thank God) triumphantly. It spared her all pain (she had no sensation, but of a great display of sky-rockets) and saved the child all mutilation. It enabled the doctors to do, as they afterwards very readily said, in ten minutes, what might otherwise have taken them an hour and a half; the shock to her nervous system was reduced to nothing; and she was, to all intents and purposes, well, next day. ... I am convinced that it is as safe in its administration, as it is miraculous and merciful in its effects.[112]

Darwin and Dickens had the clout to overrule medical fear of the risks of childbirth anaesthesia, and also the means to pay for it. Other husbands may have been equally insistent. But in the public arena doctors continued to voice their concerns. It was to fall to the best-known mother in the land to effectively silence the debate.

Queen Victoria's dislike and distaste for the states of pregnancy and childbirth was well known. From the birth of her first child, Princess Victoria, in 1840, she found pregnancy to be 'wretched': 'one becomes so worn out and one's nerves so miserable,' she wrote to the Princess when the Princess herself was pregnant in 1859. The Queen suffered from post-natal depression, particularly after her first two children, experiencing feelings of 'occasional lowness and tendency to cry'.[113] Only weeks after Simpson's discovery in November 1847, her friend Harriet, Duchess of Sutherland sent her a copy of Simpson's pamphlet. At the time the Queen was enduring her sixth pregnancy. In March 1848 she gave birth to Princess Louise after an unusually bad labour, borne without chloroform. It must have occurred to her that chloroform promised a way out of such suffering. But medical confidence had been badly shaken by the death of 15-year-old Hannah Greener three months earlier. Caution prevailed, particularly in the Royal medical household.

Sir James Clark had been Queen Victoria's physician since her succession to the throne in 1837 but almost lost his appointment in 1839 after a misdiagnosis of Lady Flora Hastings, lady-in-waiting to the Duchess of Kent, the Queen's mother. After several weeks' illness and with symptoms of pain in her left side, and swelling of her stomach, Lady Flora consulted Sir James. Gossip abounded through the Court: was the unmarried Lady Flora with child? Sir James—who had only been allowed to examine her 'over her dress'—gave credence to the rumours. To save her reputation Lady Flora submitted to a full physical examination performed by Sir James and Sir Charles Clarke, specialist in women's diseases who happened to be on hand at Buckingham Palace. The two physicians gave her a certificate: 'there are no grounds for believing pregnancy does exist, or ever had existed,' but the fallout for Sir James was considerable.[114] He was dismissed from the service of the Duchess of Kent and much pressure was put upon Queen Victoria to let him go as well. He clung to his position though his mistake lost him many patients. His reputation was damaged further when Lady Flora died only a few months later: the post-mortem showed she had suffered from liver cancer which had caused abdominal swelling. This traumatic experience may have coloured Sir James's attitude to anything new or risky. Charles Locock, appointed as Royal accoucheur in 1840, was also conservative in view and indeed, was too junior to sway Sir James's opinion on childbirth anaesthesia, even if he had wanted to.

In November 1849, three months pregnant with Prince Arthur, Queen Victoria wrote again to her friend Harriet, Duchess of Sutherland, whose daughter had just given birth using chloroform, expressing her keen interest in the matter. Later in this pregnancy she must have urged her medical advisers to let her use chloroform: they apparently raised the matter with Snow. But despite his confidence in chloroform the Royal doctors remained unconvinced. Prudence won the toss and the Queen endured a seventh labour without pain relief on 1 May 1850.

By 1852 the tide was beginning to turn. Snow was gaining Clark's and Locock's confidence. Locock recommended Snow to administer chloroform to Mrs Wood, wife of the resident medical officer at Bethlem Hospital who was suffering greatly in pregnancy. Sir James quelled his lingering doubts by watching Snow administer chloroform during the birth of Mrs Clack's first child. Prince Albert may also have swung the vote. A keen supporter of science, the Prince had become President of the new Royal College of Chemistry in 1845 and attended lectures at the Royal Institution, often given by its charismatic director, Michael Faraday, on popular topics such as electromagnetism. The Great Exhibition of 1851 had been his brainchild. He had also appointed Robinson—who carried out the first trials of ether in London—as his dentist in 1849. Perhaps the Prince had some direct experience of anaesthesia; certainly he invited Snow to the Palace sometime during March 1853. It was their first meeting and from the outset they enjoyed a good rapport. Only four years apart in age, they were both foreigners of a kind in the capital city, and shared an enthusiasm and practical interest in scientific matters. The Prince's taste for machinery of every kind gave him an ability to spot missing cogwheels in the most vast and complicated engine. As they spoke of the Queen's forthcoming labour, the Prince asking him about the scientific principles which lay behind the process of inhaling chloroform, and Snow explaining how anaesthesia affected the body's physiology, they discovered they shared a mutual interest in the new science. Snow probably explained the distinction he made between the use of chloroform for surgery and its use during childbirth: complete unconsciousness was necessary for surgery, whereas during childbirth the intention was simply to numb the pain; this did not require the patient to be totally insensible. It was particularly pertinent as yet another fatality had recently occurred at University College Hospital. Twenty-eight-year-old Caroline Baker had gone into hospital to be treated for an ulcer on her vagina but died after inhaling chloroform: 'Death was produced by a paralysis of the heart from the influence of the chloroform,' stated the inquest verdict. Prince Albert was not put off and Snow left the Palace 'much pleased' with the warmth and kindness of the meeting and impressed by the Prince's 'great intelligence on the scientific points'. [115] It was now a matter of waiting.

Receiving the Royal summons to Buckingham Palace on 7 April 1853 must have been nerve-wracking for Snow, but also thrilling. What better opportunity to silence the critics of childbirth anaesthesia than a demonstration of its safety and efficaciousness on the monarch herself? The distance from his home in Sackville Street to the Palace was less than a mile, not a long journey in a cab but time enough for Snow to consider the task before him. The Queen was desperate to benefit from chloroform, but it had taken almost six years to convince her medical entourage the risk was worth the taking. Snow's confidence in anaesthesia was supreme. But he could not have been unaware of the possible consequences—not just for himself, but also for the nation—if the birth did not proceed according to plan.

At the Palace, Snow joined Sir James and Locock in an anteroom, close to the Queen's bedroom. The three men, who by now knew each other well, waited, acutely aware of the precedent being set: Sir James and Locock trusting they had taken the right decision; Snow confident in chloroform's safety but apprehensive maybe about meeting the Queen. Whilst in the initial stages of labour, the Queen preferred to be cared for by her 'constant source of comfort and support'—Prince Albert—and Mrs Lilly, the midwife who had helped at all previous births. Around midday the Queen was coming to the end of the first stage of labour: Locock asked Snow to come through. At the bedside, Snow carefully measured out 15 minims of chloroform onto a handkerchief (a minim is equivalent to 0.06 ml), folded it into a conical shape, then held it over the Queen's mouth and nose. He was satisfied to note, 'Her Majesty expressed great relief from the application, the pains being very trifling during the uterine contractions, whilst between the periods of contractions there was complete ease.'

Prince Albert, Sir James, Locock, and Ferguson must have scrutinized Snow's every move. Locock, in particular, was edgy that chloroform might slow the labour down and delay or complicate the birth. Snow's manner at the bedside was always calm and concentrated: 'as a general rule', he often said, 'it is desirable not to hold any conversation whilst the patient is taking chloroform, in order that her mind may not be excited.' A little more chloroform was given with each pain and Prince Leopold, Duke of Albany, was born at thirteen minutes past one, according to the clock in the room. Snow, with his eye for detail, noticed that this clock was running fast—three minutes before the right time according to his watch. Once the baby was born and the placenta delivered, the Queen recovered quickly and was very cheerful, telling Snow she was most 'gratified' with the effects of the chloroform. There was delight all around, not just that the baby was born well and healthy but that the Queen's expectations of chloroform had been met. Whatever Snow's confidence in the scientific principles of inhalation, nothing was more rewarding than a grateful patient. Locock took Snow to one side: he thought 'the chloroform prolonged the interval between the pains, and retarded the labour somewhat', he said.[116] Locock had the good fortune to have already delivered seven healthy Royal babies—his fee for the first delivery was 1,000 guineas—he had, it was said, the best obstetric practice in London. He did not want to jeopardize his track record. His antipathy to chloroform can be regarded more sympathetically if we remember that it was only thirty-odd years since Princess Charlotte, daughter of King George IV and heiress to the Throne, had died in childbirth after delivering a stillborn son in 1817. Sir Richard Croft, the doctor in charge, was blamed for the tragedy: he later committed suicide.

Snow's use of the handkerchief is curious. From the first, he stressed the importance of using measured amounts of anaesthetic drugs and designed various inhalers to make sure that this could be done. 'I nearly always employ, in obstetric cases, the inhaler that I use in surgical operations … I find the inhaler much more convenient of application than a handkerchief, and it contains a supply of chloroform which lasts for some time, thereby saving the trouble of constantly pouring out more,' he wrote a few weeks after his Royal attendance.[117] Occasionally he recorded using a handkerchief in labours if the woman was distressed and not able to tolerate a face-mask. Prince Albert may have suggested that Queen Victoria would prefer to inhale chloroform from a handkerchief, or perhaps it was at Simpson's behest. Friend of Sir James and accoucheur to the Queen in Scotland, Simpson was well regarded by the Royal Household and had argued strongly for the handkerchief's superiority. Whatever the motivation, it ran against the grain of Snow's preferred way of practice and appears ironic.

Snow's skills and expertise were the safeguards on which Sir James and Locock rested their reputations. He was well chosen, not just for his skills but also for his discretion and never published one reference to his attendance upon the Queen. The only record we have of the event comes from his handwritten casebooks from the period. Not surprisingly he was often asked to spill the beans. 'Her Majesty is a model patient' was his unfailing reply. On one occasion he was giving chloroform to a 'very loquacious lady' who refused to inhale unless he told her 'what the Queen said, word for word, when she was taking it'. 'Her Majesty asked no questions until she had breathed very much longer than you have; and if you will only go on in loyal imitation, I will tell you everything,' he replied.[118] Once he had finished giving the anaesthetic he left very quickly, before the lady remembered his promise, he told his friend Richardson.

For Queen Victoria, as for Emma Darwin and Kate Dickens, chloroform transformed the experience of labour. It was 'soothing, quieting, delightful beyond measure', she wrote in her journal on 22 April 1853: never had she recovered better from a birth. Her medical advisers were swift to spread the news of the success: Sir James, effusive now that the event was over, wrote to his friend Simpson in Edinburgh; the Queen sent her own glowing report.

The usual celebrations marked Prince Leopold's birth: church bells rang throughout London, fireworks exploded over the Thames, the House of Commons sent congratulations to the Queen and Prince Albert, and the birth was announced in the national and provincial newspapers. But neither Snow nor chloroform was mentioned. The court certificate was signed only by Sir James and Locock though Snow's name was listed on the Court circular announcing the birth. Did the Palace deliberately downplay Snow's involvement? Probably not is the answer. Snow was not a member of the Royal medical household so there was neither a precedent nor a requirement for him to sign off the Court certificate. Like many other births Snow attended during 1853, he administered the chloroform and took no responsibility for the birth itself. Strict medical etiquette was applied to these situations: there was a strong demarcation between a patient's usual doctor and another who attended either as a special-ist, or to give a second opinion.

The event soon took the medical world by storm. The administra-tion of chloroform to the Queen was 'an event of unquestionable medical importance', proclaimed the editor of the *Association Medi-cal Journal* several days after the birth. Snow was a highly skilled practitioner; he affirmed and hoped the event would remove the 'lingering professional and popular prejudice against the use of an-aesthesia in midwifery'.[119] But the matter did not end here.

Almost a month later, the *Lancet* published a strong editorial re-futing the 'rumour' about the Queen's use of chloroform. 'In no case could it be justifiable to administer chloroform in perfectly ordinary labour; but the responsibility of advocating such a proceeding in the case of the Sovereign of these realms, would indeed, be tremendous.' The 'obstetric physicians to whose ability the safety of our illustrious Queen is confided do not sanction the use of chloroform in natural labour,' claimed the journal. Chloroform was of 'immense impor-tance in surgical operations', but the 'dangerous practice' of using it when it was unnecessary to do so, for example during 'a perfectly natural labour', should be soundly condemned. 'Royal examples are followed with extraordinary readiness by a certain class of society in this country,' it concluded pompously.[120]

Several questions arise. First, why did the *Lancet* take so long to run its editorial? There would have been many occasions between 7 April and 14 May when *Lancet* reporters would have been attend-ing medical society meetings. Given the involvement of Snow, Sir James and Locock, and the medical gossip network it seems un-likely the journal could have missed out on such a juicy bit of news. Second, why did the *Lancet* attempt to attribute the use of chloro-form simply to the status of malicious rumour? Thomas Wakley, the journal's editor since its inception in 1823, was deliberately provocative on many medical issues and was no supporter of Snow's theory on cholera, but it seems hardly credible that he genuinely believed the story to be false. The next mention of the Royal birth came in the *Medical Times and Gazette* on the following Saturday. It stated that it was well aware of the Queen's use of chloroform but had held back from a public announcement 'because we did not think the Profession justified in prying into the domestic arrangements of the Palace'.[121] It fully supported the use of chloroform, arguing that all mothers should have the right to benefit from chloroform's advantages. The *Association Medical Journal*, fearing that the accuracy of its reporting was being questioned, tackled the issue again on 27 May, stressing that 'chloroform during labour is entirely free from danger': it gave 'merciful relief ... in one of the most agonizing trials of humanity'.[122]

From here onwards the publicity faded. One or two provincial newspapers reprinted the story but it was soon overtaken by more pressing issues. Snow refrained from public debate and instead wrote an authoritative paper on all aspects of the administration of chloroform during childbirth. 'I believe', he said, 'the patient may be fairly allowed to have a voice in this, as in other matters of detail.' He sent it to be published in the *Association Medical Journal*—in appreciation, perhaps, of the tone of their previous editorials. Such disagreement between the leading medical journals of the day was a fair representation of the corporate views of the medical profession. Even after announcements of the Queen's use of chloroform and the publication of Snow's article, Dr Sheppard, a physician living in the provinces, felt strongly enough to write to the *Association Medical Journal* saying he would not change his view of chloroform. 'No female for whom I have any regard shall ever, with my consent, inhale chloroform,' he vowed, 'I look upon its exhibition as a pandering to the weakness of humanity, especially the weaker sex.'[123]

Some doctors agreed with Sheppard. But the Royal use of chloroform made it increasingly difficult for them to win support.

Within days of his attending Queen Victoria, some of the most influential families in the capital were calling on Snow and asking for his services. On 23 April he gave chloroform to the Honourable Mrs Proctor Beauchamp; it was her first confinement and he could see that 'the pains [were] pretty strong', so he gave chloroform 'for about the last three quarters of an hour, the inhaler being employed' and was glad to report that 'the patient went on extremely well'.[124] In the early hours of 28 April, he was called from his bed to Lady Constance Grosvenor, who lived at Stafford House (now Lancaster) in St James's Place. Built by the Duke of York around 1825, Stafford House was famous for its collection of paintings by artists such as Murillo, Van Dyck, and Moroni. As with the Queen, Snow gave Lady Constance chloroform on a handkerchief—it gave her so much relief that she slept between the contractions and 'did not complain of the pain'. Labour continued until nine in the morning when the baby was born. Snow, pleased with yet another success, declared the new mother to be 'feeling well' and 'very cheerful': chloroform had assisted the dilation of the uterus, affirmed Gream, who delivered the baby.[125] The safety and propriety of pain relief in labour was further underlined by another notable commission that autumn when Snow attended Mrs Thomas, daughter of the Archbishop of Canterbury, at Lambeth Palace.

In 1857, Snow was told that the Queen wanted to use chloroform again but before he was called to the Palace he suffered a significant blow. During 1856 he had begun to experiment with the use of amylene as an anaesthetic and was initially well pleased with the results. On 7 April 1857, expecting a summons from the Palace at any moment, he went to Regent Street with William Fergusson, by now London's premier surgeon, to operate on Mr Wellington from

Liverpool. A healthy-looking, well-made man, Wellington was 33 years old and had recently returned from Australia. He suffered from an anal fistula which had previously been repaired in 1851. The operation commenced but soon Snow noticed that 'the valve of the face-piece had moved so as to cover the aperture.'

> I discontinued the inhalation as the patient showed no sign of pain, … I began to feel for the pulse … I did not perceive it in the left wrist, and only a slight flutter in the right one. His breathing was, however, very good … there was some motion, both of his features and limbs, as if he were recovering. After two or three minutes, however, he seemed to be getting more insensible, and the breathing was getting slower and deeper. I told Mr Fergusson he was not going on well.

Fergusson was washing his hands, the operation having been concluded, and both he and Mr Price, the assistant, were very surprised that Snow thought there was a problem. Cold water was immediately dashed on Wellington's face but to no effect. By now, said Snow,

> he was … livid and the breathing of a very gasping character. The breathing left off, except deep, distant, gasping inspirations, and we performed artificial respiration, first by rolling in the method recommended by Dr Marshall Hall, then by pressing on the chest, the face being turned to one side … [we] continued for an hour and a half without effect … there was no remaining sensibility.[126]

Snow had only discovered amylene the previous year and during preliminary trials on animals found it had many positive features. Amylene was safer than chloroform, believed Snow. It was also a more pleasant anaesthetic for patients with a shorter recovery time and less sickness. Wellington was Snow's one hundred and forty-fourth amylene patient. After the post-mortem Snow attributed the cause of death to emphysema in Wellington's lungs which had in some way obstructed the pulmonary circulation: he ruled out amylene as the cause of death and continued to use it as an anaesthetic for a further ninety patients until a second fatality was to occur on 30 July. Snow then abandoned amylene and returned to chloroform.

The unexpected death of Wellington during a routine operation must have unsettled Snow. It could have made him anxious about his forthcoming attendance on the Queen, particularly as her pregnancy had been difficult. The Queen confided to Prince Albert that her physical condition caused her 'a deep sense of degradation'. Sir James had warned the Prince the previous year that the Queen was 'sure if she had another child she would sink under it': Sir James believed her mind, rather than her health, would suffer.[127] The baby was due at the beginning of April. The days passed. Snow received no call to the Palace; the Queen's medical advisers became anxious. Finally, in the early hours of a cold spring morning, 14 April, Snow was woken with a message from Sir James asking him to come at once. Arriving at Buckingham Palace he met again with Sir James and Locock but on this occasion there was a long wait in store for them. The labour appeared more difficult, the contractions were irregular, and the Queen was already suffering from the pain. After some discussion Prince Albert tried to ease this by giving her a very small amount of chloroform on a handkerchief. By ten in the morning the doctors had been there for almost eight hours; they decided to try and speed matters up. 'Locock administered half a drachm of powdered ergot, which produced some effect in increasing the pains' and 'at 11 o'clock I began to administer the chloroform' pouring 'about 10 minims of chloroform, on a handkerchief folded in a conical shape, for each pain' which gave Her Majesty 'great relief', recorded Snow. The labour progressed but the Queen 'kept asking for more chloroform, and complaining that it did not remove the pain'. When the baby was ready to be born she 'complained she could not make an effort. The chloroform was left off for 3 or 4 pains and the Royal patient made an effort which expelled the head, a little chloroform being given just as the head passed.'[128] The baby cried almost as soon as the head was born, although it was several minutes before the body followed. The Queen's spirits were immediately transformed: 'I have felt better and stronger this time than I have ever done before. I was amply rewarded and forgot all I had gone through when I heard dearest Albert say "it is a fine child, and a girl"!'[129] Four years hence, the Queen was to cling to the little Princess Beatrice for comfort after the death of Prince Albert in 1861 from typhoid. However, this was all to come and for the Queen, Beatrice's birth marked the beginning of an 'epoch' of progress. For Snow, giving chloroform to Queen Victoria again boosted his practice: during May 1857 he administered over 100 anaesthetics.

The reports of the birth of Princess Beatrice show a sea change. 'The labour was in every respect natural, as was the presentation ... the pains were somewhat lingering and ineffective' and so it was 'thought desirable that chloroform should be administered ... the anaesthetic agent perfectly succeeded in the object desired', calmly explained the *Lancet*.[130] Snow was referred to by name in the *Guardian* although there was no mention of chloroform. It had taken ten years for the use of pain relief in childbirth to be accepted as standard medical practice by even its most outspoken critics. A large part of this, certainly in London, was due to Snow's wide promotion of the practice and science of anaesthesia. It also bore testimony to patient preference for pain relief in all circumstances.

Later that year Snow was rewarded for his services to the Queen with an invitation to a levée—one of the most sought after events of the London season. Despite the Reform Bill of 1832 and the Chartist protests of the 1840s during which working-class men and women demanded universal suffrage, the Court was still seen as the pinnacle of British society. Levées were strictly male-only events and were packed with the aristocracy, government ministers, and the highest ranking officers from the armed forces: ladies made their Court appearances at Drawing Room events. Sponsors forwarded recommendations to the Lord Chamberlain: in Snow's case, Sir James asked for him to be put on the list.

So on 18 June 1857 Snow set out for St James's Palace, the oldest of the London royal establishments—this time without chloroform. A Royal presentation took a matter of seconds but carried a huge mark of prestige within the highest ranks of society. Receiving up to five hundred presentees was a hot and exhausting business for the Queen; she was always grateful when the series came to a close each year. But she had a genuine warmth and gratitude for Snow's administration of 'that blessed chloroform'. Whether it occurred to Snow as he knelt before her that the Queen was in a more composed and dignified state than in their previous encounters is left to conjecture.

Princess Beatrice was the last child of the Queen and Prince Albert. Nevertheless Royal mothers continued to benefit from chloroform. Sir James attended Princess Victoria, the Empress Frederick, at the birth of her first child in January 1859 in Berlin. The Queen was prevented from attending because of the opening of Parliament so, in her lieu, she sent Sir James, Mrs Innocent, her midwife, and a bottle of chloroform. Only just over a year later, in the summer of 1860, Princess Vicky was expecting her second child. She asked Sir James to send a bottle of chloroform directly to her with instructions to the Court doctor that she should be given enough of it. 'Last time what little I got I owe to good Sir James who held it to my nose in spite of Wegner (the court doctor) … here you know they have such different ideas on that subject,' she told the Queen. The birth was 'much easier' than Wilhelm's and Princess Charlotte was born on 24 July. Princess Alice, the Queen's third child, was given chloroform freely during the last ninety minutes of the birth of her first child on 8 April 1863. Later that same year in July, Marie, wife of Prince Alfred, underwent 'an awful labour', said the Queen: '48 hours in pain and 18 in constant labour! I sat by her and they put her completely under chloroform and she was like as if she slept, I stroking her face all the time and while Dr Farre most skilfully and cleverly delivered her without her knowing or feeling anything, and only woke when she heard the child cry.' [131]

Snow played no part in these Royal births: he had died suddenly in June 1858 aged only 45 years. But his skill and confidence in anaesthesia and the Queen's tenacity in seeking pain relief in childbirth was a winning combination: 'chloroform à la reine' put the seal of respectability on childbirth anaesthesia.

5

. . . .

ON BATTLEFIELDS

On 28 February 1854, with the sun rising over the towers of Westminster Abbey, Queen Victoria stood on the balcony at Buckingham Palace and watched the last battalion of the Guards— the Scots Fusiliers regiment—depart for the Crimea. Engulfed by an immense crowd shouting encouragements and shaking their hands, the men formed a line, presented arms, and went off cheering. Such 'fine men', the Queen told her uncle, King Leopold I of Belgium, 'my best wishes and prayers will be with them'.[132] *The Times* correspondent who watched the 30,000 or so troops embark at Portsmouth en route for the Baltic echoed her thoughts: 'the finest army that ever left these shores.' But the Crimean War was to result in the death of half a million men. It was provoked by Russia's invasion of Turkish provinces in the Balkans in 1853. Britain, concerned about Russia's growing power, supported Turkey and, in alliance with France, declared war on Russia. The war and its causes, said Frederick Engels, 'was a colossal comedy of errors'. The twentieth-century historian E. J. Hobsbawm described it as an event of 'notoriously incompetent international butchery'.[133]

Britain had enjoyed almost forty years of peace since the Napoleonic wars. By the 1850s daily life had been transformed by a huge range of innovations: steam railways, the penny post, and the electric telegraph to name but a few. The electric telegraph in particular revolutionized communication links between Britain and her fighting forces in the Crimea. One of the first tasks undertaken by British troops at the beginning of the war was to lay a telegraph line across the Black Sea to the eastern shore, the site of early conflicts: the word 'telegram' entered British vocabulary. The Crimean War was the first war to be fought in the fierce glare of public interest, fanned by widespread coverage in newspapers and journals. Despatches from war correspondents, living and travelling with the troops, pulled no punches in telling the public exactly what conditions were like: their reports appeared in Britain within days. Indeed, the frequent and detailed accounts sent home by William Howard Russell, correspondent to *The Times*, caused one Russian to declare, 'we have no need of spies we have the *Times*'.[134] Through the new medium of photography Roger Fenton captured images of troops handling a new generation of weaponry. Muskets which fired balls had been forsaken for the 'Enfield Rifle', a British modification of the French Minie rifle, which fired a cartridge. It swiftly became standard army issue but for those caught in its fire: 'the tissues were more injured, the bone more shattered, and the suppuration more profuse', explained Thomas Burgess, who treated gunshot wounds at the military hospital in Portsmouth.[135] New technology created submarines and devices which promised to subdue high waves at sea and enable ships to land during storms. Whilst soldiers fought on the battlefields of the Crimea, battles raged amongst doctors seeking to resolve controversies about the risks and benefits of anaesthesia for severely wounded soldiers.

The launch missile came in a warning to medical officers by inspector general of hospitals and chief medical officer Sir John Hall. Extreme caution was to be exercised about the use of chloroform when treating battle injuries, particularly amputations resulting from gunshot wounds: remember the 'smart of the knife is a powerful stimulant and it is much better to hear a man bawl lustily than to see him sink silently into the grave', Hall told his officers in September 1854.[136] He knew his words would appear barbaric to the public, but was adamant that soldiers suffering shock from severe wounds would not survive under chloroform. The *Instructions to Troops* were reprinted in the *Illustrated London News* and opened the floodgates to a welter of argument and condemnation. Buoyed up by the strong sense of national pride it probably seemed outrageous to those who read his message that soldiers wounded whilst fighting for their country would not be treated as humanely as possible. But Hall's concerns about the risks of chloroform were genuine and plagued many of his fellow doctors at the time.

A veteran of Waterloo, Hall was a strong medical conservative. His views on anaesthetics reflected his age. Hall viewed pain as a benefit and physiological necessity: pain was a stimulant during an operation. Other veteran surgeons like George Guthrie were equally cautious. Anaesthesia was believed to act as a depressant and compound the risks of surgery: in short, to raise the stakes of death. Shocked or severely wounded soldiers were thought most vulnerable to the dangers of chloroform. Shock, usually from major blood loss rather than circulatory, or psychological causes was a recognized phenomenon in civilian casualties, particularly railway or industrial accidents. What seemed to exacerbate 'shock' on the battlefield was that fighting soldiers were pushed to their physical and mental limits at the time of the injury. This heightened state—today we would talk about a rush of adrenalin through the body—seemed to intensify the reaction of the nervous system to the injury. The wounded lapsed into a period of stupor, seemingly hovering on the fringes of death. Medical decisions pivoted on balancing the risk of operating immediately, perhaps whilst the injured man was protected by the stupor, or postponing surgery until consciousness was regained. In such fraught circumstances pain seemed to help save lives. But the younger generation saw pain in a new way. Only months after the introduction of ether, John Snow told military doctors of the benefits anaesthesia brought to wounded soldiers:

> A great part of the danger of an operation consists in the pain of it, which gives a shock to the system from which it is sometimes unable to recover. If an operation is performed during or immediately after an action, the wounded man suffers two shocks together—that of his wound and that of the operation, which although, singly, his frame might sustain, united, perhaps it cannot. If on the other hand, a secondary operation ... has to be performed sometime afterwards ... he is rendered more susceptible of pain by his illness and suffering ... I believe that ether will give the surgeon a greater choice in selecting between cases for immediate and subsequent operation, for dread of the knife helps to cause and keep up the faintness and collapse, which will often prevent the surgeon from operating at once.[137]

Few were as sure as Snow of the benefits. In the 1840s most doctors used anaesthetics sparingly in military conflict. The first occasion ether was used in war was during the USA conflict with Mexico in 1847. Texas had declared independence from Mexico in 1835 and was admitted into the USA in 1845. Conflict ensued and war broke out between the USA and Mexico in May 1846, continuing through the autumn whilst William Morton was establishing ether in Boston. By 1847 US forces were fighting in Vera Cruz. Morton, ever swift to spot a financial opportunity, approached the US military. The new anaesthetic—ether—could benefit 'suffering soldiers and sailors in the Mexican War', he suggested, and promised the US Navy and the Surgeon General of the US Army that he could despatch agents to Mexico at once: 'the expense to the Government would only be but a few hundred dollars'; the cost of apparatus would be knocked down to wholesale prices, he cajoled. His offer was rejected but ether was used.

Edward H. Barton, surgeon to the Third Dragoons of the Cavalry Brigade of Twigg's division, was in the fleet which blockaded the port of Vera Cruz. Barton had set off for war taking a supply of ether and an apparatus. After a difficult first attempt at administering the ether, Barton succeeded in removing a soldier's limb 'without the quiver of a muscle'. Mexican soldiers wounded in the fighting were not so fortunate. Whilst they were operated on, officers ordered the military band to play so as to drown out the sounds of their 'lamentations'. But Surgeon General of the US army, John B. Porter, ruled that ether was too risky: it could cause haemorrhage, blood poisoning, and even gangrene, and was 'a decidedly unfavourable influence upon the state of the wounds and upon the result of the operation'.[138] Opponents to anaesthesia latched onto Porter's views and he was quoted across Britain and Europe.

But in the same year Russian soldiers did benefit from ether, thanks to the surgeon Nikolai Ivanovich Pirogoff, professor at the Military Medico-Surgical Academy in St Petersburg. Pirogoff took up ether as soon as news reached him early in 1847: he is known in anaesthetic history for pioneering rectal administration of ether—a particularly useful method of administration for the very painful and most serious operations, he noted. Only months later he departed to Piatigorsk to care for Russian soldiers fighting rebels in the Caucasus region. One hundred wounded soldiers were given ether and some operations were performed on the battlefield. Pirogoff's experience was to stand him in good stead for the Crimean War.

Russia was not the only nation to experience civil uprisings during the late 1840s. Across Europe, poor potato and wheat harvests provoked unrest. Riots on the streets of Paris, resulting in more than a thousand deaths and many thousands more injuries, marked the beginning of a wave of protest that swept through Austria-Hungary, Italy, and Germany between 1848 and 1852. Surgeons treating the injured faced the most serious challenge of all: gunshot wounds. The musket balls were 'propelled with such force and velocity, that they will divide vessels and nerves, and shatter bones into pieces', Louis Velpeau, Professor of Surgery in Paris told his students.[139] Immediate amputation was the only solution, preferably whilst the patient was still in a state of stupor caused by the shock of the injury. But some patients resisted the loss of a limb. On 24 February 1848, at the height of the riots, one poor man had his arm fractured by a musket ball; he refused to submit to an amputation, as did another whose leg and knee had been shattered, again by a musket ball. Velpeau only gained their consent for an operation several days after the initial injuries. But he did not use chloroform for such patients—it depresses the nervous system and compounds the prostration, he argued—though patients with lesser injuries benefited: doctor and reporter Charles Kidd, sent to Paris by the *Medical Times,* watched Velpeau and his colleagues carry out around 1,600 operations under chloroform in the wake of the riots.

Like Velpeau, John Jones Cole, surgeon to the auxiliary forces in the Punjab, resisted the use of anaesthetics because of the powerful stimulant nature of pain. Cole set up a hospital in Mooltan to treat casualties of the second Sikh war in 1848–9 which had been provoked by the occupation of the Punjab by the British East India Company. Examining one of the amputees, Cole congratulated his fellow surgeon: 'a better or cleaner stump I have not often noticed.' But, he warned, 'you will not ... save your patient ... he looks as if he had taken chloroform.' 'We did give him chloroform and he did not suffer the slightest pain,' retorted his colleague.[140] Cole's prophecy of doom was fulfilled: the patient died before evening.

Nevertheless, some doctors persisted in using chloroform for British and native casualties. William Barker M'Egan, assistant surgeon to his Highness the Nizam's second regiment of cavalry Mominabad, praised the benefits of anaesthesia in a letter to the *Lancet*: 'I never found any bad effects to follow.'[141] Out of forty-nine injured natives, forty-six recovered following operations under chloroform and returned to battle, claimed M'Egan. In keeping with ideas about supposed differentiated sensibility of different races, M'Egan had assumed that the natives (with less sensibility) would be less susceptible to chloroform's effects. Instead they were as receptive as British soldiers. A later report of the campaign tempered M'Egan's buoyant account, suggesting that there was a higher mortality amongst the fifty-three patients operated on under chloroform than among the forty-seven patients who had endured surgery without pain relief.

By the early 1850s anaesthesia had proved itself to be beneficial in war, though surgeons remained wary about its use. Hall's caution on the use of chloroform infuriated many doctors, particularly the Scottish medical clans. North of the English border, chloroform was used routinely in surgery. Edinburgh's discoverer James Simpson urged doctors setting out for war to take a bottle with them. His colleague James Syme opposed Hall's views in a letter to *The Times*: 'chloroform does not increase the danger of operations performed during a state of exhaustion, however extreme … pain instead of being a "powerful stimulant" most injuriously exhausts the nervous energy of a weak patient,' he remonstrated.[142] Other writers supported Syme's arguments but news of a chloroform fatality at University College Hospital, London, seemed further proof of its dangers. Whilst words were being bandied in the columns of *The Times*, allied forces in the Crimea were seeking to capture and destroy the Russian naval port at Sebastopol. During the first battle, fought on top of the precipitous cliffs fringing the river Alma, injured soldiers were given chloroform by Richard Mackenzie, one of Simpson's protégés who had rapidly dismissed Hall's dictum: 'Dr Hall's order is to discourage the use of it altogether. No one, I think should take any notice of it.'[143] Mackenzie's service was short: he died from cholera a few days after the conflict in October 1854. Only weeks later, the first soldier died after chloroform.

On 5 November 1854 in the hills surrounding the Sebastopol, the 'memorable and bloody' battle of Inkerman was fought. The British suffered 2,357 casualties, one of whom was a 29-year-old soldier who suffered a compound fracture of his femur, lost much blood on the field, and pleaded for chloroform during the operation. His wish was granted but he died suddenly after surgery. Chloroform administrator James Mouat, who later won the Victoria Cross at Balakclava, was convinced that the soldier's death was caused by 'the combined influence of shock and the depressing effects of the chloroform'.[144] More fortunate was Mark Walker: he survived the amputation of his arm under chloroform, and won the Victoria Cross for bravery. He wrote in his journal,

> While I was in the act of hurrying the men up, a howeitzer shell dropped beside me and exploded. A piece struck me on the right elbow and smashed it. I immediately tied a large handkerchief above the fracture and walked to the rear until I met some of the 55th who put me on a stretcher and carried me to Camp. I received great kindness from my new brother officers. After some time I was carried to a hut at the General Hospital where I now am. I was put under chloroform and on coming to consciousness I found my arm taken off above the elbow during the night and today I suffered a good deal of pain. The loss I have experienced is very great but I am very thankful that my life has been spared. The hut has been filled with sympathising visitors particularly my old comrades of the 30th.[145]

The great change in handwriting between earlier entries and this one poignantly expresses his loss.

In the base hospitals chloroform was in regular use. 'Chloroform was always used' in Scutari, even though there was no operating table, reported the Revd Sydney Osborne, almoner to *The Times* Crimean fund in November 1854.[146] Surgeon George Pyemount Smith confirmed this:

> I had been accustomed to the use of chloroform, but certainly had never seen it given to the extent that it was employed here ... at Scutari, the patient was, by means of chloroform, brought into the condition of a dead body, and then it was not an operation, but a dissection that was performed.[147]

But chloroform use was often curtailed more through a lack of supplies than by theoretical arguments.

Regimental surgeons were initially issued with 8 oz of chloroform in their field panniers—enough to cover between four and six major operations. The distribution of chloroform amongst the different divisions and regiments was patchy. At the battle of Alma, whereas the 88th regiment which suffered 17 wounded men had 2 lb 8 oz of chloroform at their disposal, no chloroform was available for the 7th Fusiliers who sustained 179 wounded soldiers. Out of the eleven ships used to transport the wounded from the Crimea to the hospital in Scutari during September 1854, only two had substantial supplies of chloroform on board. As the ships wended their way across the sea to Scutari, surgeons worked ceaselessly. But the lack of chloroform meant that few soldiers had pain relief. The *Colombo* carried 650 officers and men wounded in the battle of Alma: 'Nothing but cutting off arms and legs all day long ... we could not work fast enough to save all the wounded on board. I had one amputation of the shoulder-joint, and as for thighs and legs, I left off counting them,' recalled one of the surgeons.[148] The ship's 'decks

were running with blood the whole time worse than shambles, and
the exhalations were overpowering in the extreme,' according to
another officer.[149] Lack of manpower, particularly in the midst of
battle, also compromised the use of chloroform: 'I hear there is a
great cry against our not using chloroform,' one artillery surgeon
told the *Medical Times and Gazette* after the battle of Inkerman,
'but ... it reduces the number of medical men available for duty ...
seldom can you get more than one doctor to assist at an operation
... Operating in the field and in a well-found Hospital are vastly
different affairs.'[150] Fears that chloroform would prove as inflammable as ether also caused surgeons to desist: 'We had so much smoke
and heated atmosphere from our lamps and candles and the smoke
occasionally after gunpowder, that we did not deem it advisable to
employ it [chloroform] until the action was nearly over,' explained
naval surgeon George MacKay.[151]

In contrast to the wider problems of medical services during the
war, disputes over chloroform seemed trivial. Reports of the 'glori-
ous' success at the battle of Alma made headline news in October
1854. Days later, the British public was alerted to the true state of
affairs when Thomas Chenery wrote in *The Times*:

> [I]t is with feelings of surprise and anger that the public will learn
> that no sufficient medical preparations have been made for the
> proper care of the wounded. Not only are there not sufficient sur-
> geons—that, it might be urged, was unavoidable—not only are
> there no dressers and nurses—that might be a defect of system for
> which no one is to blame—but what will be said when it is known
> that there is not even linen to make bandages for the wounded? ...
> there is no preparation for the commonest of surgical operations!
> Not only are men kept, in some cases, for a week without the hand
> of a medical man coming near their wounds; not only are they left
> to expire in agony, unheeded and shaken off, though catching des-
> perately at the surgeon whenever he makes his rounds through the

fetid ship, but now ... [it] is found that the commonest appliances of a workhouse sick-ward are wanting.

Worst of all perhaps, in terms of national pride, was the contrast with French medical services: 'their ... arrangements are extremely good, their surgeons more numerous, and they have also the help of the Sisters of Charity, ... excellent nurses.' [152] This blunt summary caught the public's imagination. 'Why have we no sisters of charity?', implored a 'Sufferer by the Present War' the following day. It also drew the attention of Florence Nightingale, superintendent of the Hospital for Invalid Gentlewomen in Harley Street to whom the difficulties in the Crimea seemed a heaven-sent opportunity.

From an early age, Nightingale was driven by a need to perform constructive activities like visiting the sick, rather than submitting to the social round. Victorian women were in danger of going mad for 'want of something to do', she said. The Nightingale family were Unitarians and Nightingale's spiritual experiences convinced her that God wanted her to work in hospitals. Her close friendship with Sydney Herbert, second son of the Earl of Pembroke, and his wife, Elizabeth, began in 1847. It was to prove the entrée to fulfilling her ambitions. In August 1853, after recommendation by Elizabeth Herbert, Nightingale became superintendent to a charitable institution in Harley Street which cared for sick governesses. Her duties included supervising supplies and services and she made many improvements. But by October 1854 she was ready for a new challenge. Her objective was to set up a nursing school in one of the London teaching hospitals; she was in discussion with King's College Hospital when the war began.

The idea of sending nurses to staff the hospitals in the Crimean had been mooted at Government level before the army left the country. But the notion received short shrift from the military. Nevertheless, the early reports in *The Times* of the appalling conditions and disorganization could not be ignored. Sydney Herbert was instrumental in the Government's decision to ask Nightingale to head up a party of nurses. He was convinced that she was the only possible candidate with the strength of character to exert moral discipline upon a group of nurses. Herbert was also aware of the wider implications of the experiment. If it was successful, he wrote, then 'a prejudice will have been broken through, & a precedent established, which will multiply the good to all time'.[153]

Nightingale and her party of nurses arrived at the English base in Scutari on 4 November 1854 where a hospital had been contrived from the old Turkish barracks.

Standing on the wooded clifftops above the Bosphorus, the hospital enjoyed magnificent views across to the domes and minarets of Constantinople and down the strait to the Golden Horn. But conditions inside the buildings were horrific. Floors were made of broken stone tiles resting upon rotten wood; windows were small and stuffed with cloth to keep out the cold; straw-filled mattresses

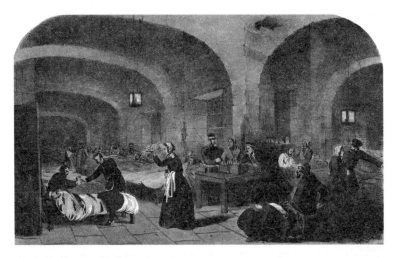

Figure 9 Florence Nightingale at Scutari.

packed the wards and the corridors. 'This is the Kingdom of Hell ...
We have not an average of three limbs per man ... operations ... are
all performed in the wards ... we have not a basin nor a towel nor a
bit of soap nor a broom,' wrote Nightingale after receiving 570 soldiers wounded in the battle of Balaclava, infamous for the Charge of
the Light Brigade—the military mayhem which sent British troops
charging into a valley surrounded by Russian artillery.[154] Nightingale immediately ordered 300 scrubbing brushes. But problems
with supplies continued to hamper medical services. Only days after
Nightingale's arrival at Scutari, a hurricane in the Black Sea sank the
steamship the *Great Britain* and its cargo of winter clothing for the
army and medical supplies. W. H. Russell reported to *The Times*:
'nearly one half of our cavalry horses broke loose. The wounded had
to bear the inclemency of the weather as best they could. ... Sleet
fell at first, then Crimea snow storm, which clothed the desolate
landscape in white, till the tramp of men seamed it with trails of
black mud.' Tales abounded of disasters: supplies arriving in Varna
after the army had departed; shipments sent to the Crimea rather
than Constantinople; some supplies were even returned to Britain;
and by November 1854 the Russians had captured the road leading
to the British camp from the harbour in Scutari and the only route
for supplies was over muddy mountain tracks.

Young military surgeons like Edward Wrench, trained at St
Thomas's Hospital in the early 1850s, were horrified by the condi-
tions. Wrench's first posting was to the British military hospital in
Balaclava which admitted men wounded at the battle of Inkerman.

> I had charge of from 20 to 30 patients, wounded from Inkerman,
> mixed with cases of cholera, dysentery, and fever. There were no beds
> ... or proper bedding. The patients lay in their clothes on the floor,
> which from rain blown in through the open windows, and the traffic
> to and from the open-air latrines, was as muddy as a country road.

Here, military use of chloroform did seem to have been tempered by Hall's edict: 'we ... only used chloroform for the more serious operations, and never to facilitate examination or for what we considered trivial operations, as cutting out bullets or setting fractures,' he recalled almost fifty years after event.[155]

'The mighty Thor, with his crown of ice', has conquered English, French, and Russian troops alike, reported the *Lancet* in January 1855. Sanitary conditions of hospitals, barracks, and battlefields allowed disease to thrive. In one instance, the soldiers' drinking water had flowed over corpses and was contaminated with excrement from the troops and animals: Snow identified impure water as the source of a cholera outbreak in Scutari. Corpses were left to rot: the image of 'dead Russians on the field of Inkerman with the crocuses blooming between their mummified fingers after the fleshy parts of the body had been devoured by birds and beasts' remained fixed in surgeon Edward Wrench's memory. Regiments were devastated by disease rather than injury. Out of the 850 men of the 46th regiment, only 70 were fit to fight. Diarrhoea headed the list of diseases suffered by inmates at Scutari hospital which included dysentery, fevers, and scurvy. The cases of frostbitten feet which arrived were 'altogether the most wretched and miserable appearance it has even been my fate to observe', exclaimed surgeon George Pyemont Smith. It was not so much the cold, but rather 'scurvy, deficient food, want of cleanliness, and long-continued exposure, without means of changing or drying the clothes when they became wet' that had reduced the men to such a low point that their extremities froze immediately the temperature dropped.[156] The *Lancet* was quick to point out that the well-fed and free from scurvy Russian troops easily withstood the same conditions. Soldiers shipped home to the military hospital in Portsmouth arrived in a deplorable state. 'Their wretched aspect, broken constitutions, emaciated frames, decrepid and aged appearance' told of their depletion by dysentery, said receiving surgeon Thomas Burgess: 'Boys of eighteen bore the haggard, time-worn aspect of men of seventy or eighty, with sunken, glazed eyes, prominent jaws, and an expression of utter prostration, painful to look at. Their bodies were crawling with vermin, and the skin encrusted with filth, and even human excrement.'[157]

British medical services were highly criticized both during and after the war but amongst the chaos of fighting and disease there were a few chinks of light as British surgeons had the opportunity to observe and, perhaps, to learn from the French and Russian forces. French surgical opinion on the risks of anaesthesia had changed since 1848 when Velpeau refrained from using chloroform for the most severely wounded. During the Crimean War, French surgeons employed chloroform without restriction, according to a protocol developed by surgeon general Gaspard Scrive: *chloroformisation de charité* sedated or gave pain relief to the dying; *chloroformisation de nécessité* was given for amputations, or extraction of bullets or other missiles; *chloroformisation de prudence* numbed patients to the pain of dressing large wounds. Scrive avoided chloroform overdosage by using the Charrière device—an inhaler which had a tap to control the concentration of chloroform—and ensuring that patients were not put into 'deep' anaesthesia. Other French surgeons relied on the simpler method of dropping chloroform on to a pasteboard cone which fitted over the patient's mouth and nose. Mounier, who served as surgeon-in-chief of Dolma Bagtche Hospital at Constantinople, claimed success 'several thousands of times'. Out of 'all the wounded of Alma and Inkerman brought to my hospital ... we have never had a death or even an accident,' he stressed.[158] During the war the French gave over 25,000 chloroform administrations seemingly without any fatalities. It was just cause for Gallic pride. At this time the mortality rate for chloroform anaesthesia in Britain was around one death in every 2,500 or so administrations. Mounier also taught chloroform administration to Turkish medical students, and encouraged them to practice surgical techniques on corpses. After the war, the Turks honoured British physician Dr Charles Johnson with a medal of the fifth degree from the Ottoman state for successfully anaesthetizing wounded soldiers in Istanbul with a mixture of ether and chloroform.

Russian medical services were headed by Pirogoff, who had used ether during warfare in 1847. His confidence in chloroform was absolute. Russian soldiers were given it for all amputations, as well as wound dressing. But not even anaesthesia could save soldiers from all suffering. Leo Tolstoy was a young artillery officer during the Crimean War and captured its sights and sounds in a series of articles for the independent newspaper, the *Russian Veteran*. The truth of war was blood, suffering, and death, he wrote after witnessing

> surgeons with pale, gloomy physiognomies, their arms soaked in blood up to their elbows, deep in concentration over a bed on which a wounded man is lying under the influence of chloroform, open-eyed as in a delirium, and uttering meaningless words which are occasionally simple and affecting. ... [Y]ou will see the sharp, curved knife enter the white, healthy body; you will see the wounded man suddenly regain consciousness with a terrible, harrowing shrieked cursing; you will see the apothecary assistant fling the severed arm into a corner.[159]

Russian surgeons were also amazed to find that they needed to give French prisoners of war twice or three times the usual amount of chloroform to achieve insensibility. Fear, it seemed, intensified pain.

By the close of the war the pendulum had swung in favour of chloroform for severely wounded soldiers. British military experience of anaesthesia was dissected by the Crimean Medical and Surgical Society. Chaired by Hall who had been knighted for his war efforts, the Society agreed that chloroform was generally beneficial. A new raft of surgical manuals published in the late 1850s distilled the experience of Crimean surgeons like Edinburgh-trained George Macleod, who served at Sebastopol. Chloroform, said Macleod, was 'of inestimable value' and pain relief could boost the morale of troops: 'much is gained in field practice by the mere avoidance of the patient's screams when undergoing operation, as it frequently happens that but a thin partition, a blanket or a few planks, intervene between him who is being operated upon, and those who wait to undergo a like trial.'[160] Even old-timers like George Guthrie, originally cautious about the use of chloroform, added an addendum to his military textbook: anaesthesia 'will always prove advantageous'.[161] Guthrie also invited Snow to draw up the principles of chloroform administration which Guthrie then taught to medical students at St George's hospital:

> Chloroform may be given with safety and advantage to every patient who requires, and is in a condition to undergo, a surgical operation. A state of great depression, from injury or disease, does not contraindicate the use of chloroform. This agent acts as a stimulant, in the first instance, increasing the strength of the pulse, and enabling the patient, in a state of exhaustion, to go through an operation much better than if he were conscious.[162]

Hall's 1854 warning on the perils of chloroform seemed a thing of the past, though military anaesthesia continued to be problematic.

Whereas the Crimean War had marked a new era of warfare in Europe, the American Civil War of 1861–5 broke new records in US military history. More than 2,000 battles were fought and around 560,000 troops lost their lives. We have good knowledge of the details of the war through the six volumes of the *Medical and Surgical History of the War of the Rebellion*, which was published by the Surgeon General's office. Most Confederate and Union surgeons agreed about the use of anaesthesia. 'The universal use of chloroform to allay the pain of surgical operations, is a complete vindication of the utility of the remedy, and proof of its necessity. ... We do not hesitate to say, that it should be given to every patient requiring a serious or painful operation,' wrote J. Julian Chisholm, Professor of Surgery in the Medical College of South Carolina, in the Confederate army manual. Chisholm, who headed the Confederate medical department and administered over 10,000 anaesthetics himself, continued: 'death sometimes ensues from nervous exhaustion, produced by excess of suffering; the use of chloroform relieves the patient at least from this risk.'[163] During the war, around 80,000 cases were treated under anaesthesia, and chloroform was the most-favoured anaesthetic. Statistics suggest that casualties of the Civil war fared marginally better than those of the Crimean War. Union surgeons had a fatality rate of 26 per cent out of 30,000 amputations; in the Crimea, the fatality rate was 28 per cent out of 1,027 amputations. Indeed, the statistics are even more persuasive in the case of amputations at the hip—the most dangerous of all amputations. Whereas all British soldiers died after this operation, 17 per cent of Civil War casualties survived. But, again, the practical difficulties of supply and demand hampered the use of anaesthetics.

The Union blockade of all southern ports in May 1861 prevented most international shipments reaching Confederate troops, and later that year not even port-to-port traffic was able to break the hold. Aside from the obvious difficulties of limiting food and clothing supplies, the blockage also prevented stocks of chloroform reaching the south. The problems were exacerbated because most of the manufacturers of chloroform were based in the northern states. Union supply trains were raided for food and chloroform, most notably by General Thomas Jonathan Jackson and his troops. In May

1862 during the battle of Winchester, Jackson—known as Stone-wall—and his party succeeded in capturing 15,000 cases of chloroform as well as other medical supplies. It was one of many successes. A year later, Jackson experienced the benefits of chloroform for himself. Shot accidentally by his own men, he breathed chloroform as his fractured arm was repaired, and sank into oblivion muttering, 'What an infinite blessing ... blessing ... blessing'. On regaining consciousness he described it as 'the most delightful physical sensation I ever experienced ... the most delightful music that ever greeted my ears', but later died from his injuries.[164]

Distribution of supplies was not the only matter of concern. Surgical inexperience was also cause for alarm. Many of the surgeon volunteers had never watched a major amputation, nor treated gunshot wounds. Not surprisingly, some were tempted to treat injuries as conservatively as possible. But often, operations afforded the only chance of recovery, argued William M. Caniff, Professor of Surgery at Toronto's University of Victoria College, who visited the Union army in the winter of 1862–3. William Williams Keen, a medical student who treated the injured, confirmed this view: 'I have no hesitation in saying that far more lives were lost in refusal to amputate than by amputation.'[165] Over-enthusiasm could be equally dangerous. At the beginning of the war 'the limbs of soldiers were in as much danger from the ardor of young surgeons as from the missiles of the enemy', noted Chisholm in his *Manual of Military Surgery*. To operate, or not to operate? To amputate or to excise? These were the questions that dominated military medical society meetings during the conflict. Amputation was the speediest option; excisions took longer and increased the anaesthetic risk. It was a decision that had untold ramifications. Edward Wrench, surgeon in the Crimea explained:

[N]o arm is much better for a soldier than an arm of little use, for the first he gets a shilling a day pension (for the loss of a limb) whereas for the latter he gets nothing, but is just turned out as unfit for service, so that the old story of where in doubt operate, is doubly applicable in the army.[166]

From 1863 onwards the US Sanitary Commission sought to eliminate such problems by establishing regulations and standards. Both Union and Confederate leaders introduced systems to ensure surgeons with the greatest experience acted as arbitrators over the decision to operate. With regard to anaesthetics, each hospital should give authority over the use of anaesthetics to one assistant surgeon, advised Jonathan Letterman, Medical Director of the Army of the Potomac. One familiar and experienced figure on the battlefield was William Morton, who gave anaesthetics to the wounded after the battles of Fredericksburg (December 1862) and Wilderness (May 1864).

Out of the 560,000 deaths which occurred during the Civil War two-thirds were caused by disease, one-third by injury. As in the Crimean War unsanitary conditions and a restricted diet, consisting mainly of hard tack biscuits and black coffee, led to much suffering. Most soldiers suffered chronic diarrhoea—it was the cause of more deaths than any other disease. No Confederate soldier had a fully formed stool for the duration of the war, recollected one physician. Scurvy and pellagra, which caused itchy skin, dementia, diarrhoea, and, ultimately, death, were common complaints. It is hardly surprising that the incidence of malingering—contriving an honourable discharge—rose rapidly.

Malingering was not a new phenomenon of war. George Guthrie, British Deputy-Inspector of Military Hospitals during the Napoleonic wars, described how a soldier had swallowed a cork full of pins to produce bloody spit. Napoleon's troops were known to push the testes of cocks and the kidneys of hares into their noses in order to pretend polyps. But most common were simulations of lameness, paralysis, deafness, blindness, and epilepsy. For those who succeeded, the benefits could be good: disability pensions or, for the Civil War malingerers, the retention of the $300 bounty paid upon conscription. Anaesthesia became a new weapon in the battle against military malingering. 'It is humiliating to the medical officer, and a loss to the country, for him to be deceived by a man who is only pretending illness; yet … the difficulties of distinguishing between real and pretended disease are sometimes very great. … Ether has solved the difficulty,' Snow confidently told a gathering of military medical officers in May 1847 and explained how under ether it was not possible to feign disabilities or deformity.[167] By the 1860s Union and Confederate surgical manuals urged surgeons to use anaesthetics to detect malingering. In Philadelphia, the hospital originally established for 'shock' victims became a specialist centre for such cases. The neurologist Silas Weir Mitchell and doctors William Williams Keen and George Morehouse placed malingerers in a state of light anaesthesia and subjected them to a plethora of physical and mental tests. Snow's view was that the benefit of doubt should be given to the soldier. By the 1860s malingerers were given no slack. In the absence of a convincing diagnosis surgeons were obliged to enforce strict criteria. 'It is hard to force a sick man to duty,' noted Chisholm. A truly sick soldier 'is pretty sure to find his way into a hospital again', William Keen reassured himself.[168] Only in the 1880s did the concept of traumatic or post-traumatic neurosis become established as a medical category of disease. By the First World War, electric shock treatment had replaced anaesthetics: 'a very strong faradic current', or even the suggestion of its forcible application, was 'almost infallible', claimed medical experts.

Military practice was also built around ideas of masculine heroic fortitude. Leaders like John B. Porter drew on notions of heroism and male stoicism in defence of their antagonism towards ether in the late 1840s. Do not confound 'the complaint of the slim soft-fibred man-milliner, with that of the firm and brawny ploughman', naval surgeon Thomas Trotter had advised in the early 1800s.[169] These ideas echoed in the reports of operations without pain relief on 254 wounded soldiers following the battle of Iuka, Mississippi, in September 1862: 'not a groan or sign of pain was heard.'[170] But generally public and medical tolerance of needless physical pain was waning fast. Chisolm chided surgeons who 'moralize upon the duty of suffering'.[171] Silas Mitchell performed experimental operations on wounded soldiers to try and relieve chronic pain in non-terminal illnesses. And anaesthesia's humane influence upon surgery boosted the integration of nursing with military medicine by making more palatable the blood and gore of war and its injuries to feminine sensibilities.

Louisa May Alcott, later famous for *Little Women*, her story of the Brookes family during the Civil War, worked as a volunteer nurse at the Union Hospital Hotel in Georgetown, Virginia. The 'enthusiasm' with which Dr P. set about investigating injuries without anaesthetics 'convinced me that I was a weaker vessel, though nothing would have induced me to confess it then', she later admitted in *Sketches of Hospital Practice*. Dr P. had served during the Crimean War and relished his work: 'the more intricate the wound, the better he liked it.' Watching him 'poke about among bits of bone and visible muscles, in a red and black chasm made by some infernal machine of the shot or shell', Alcott strongly desired 'to insinuate a few of his own disagreeable knives and scissors into him, and see how he liked it'. She reassured fellow nurses that witnessing amputations should not be part of their duties unless they so wished.

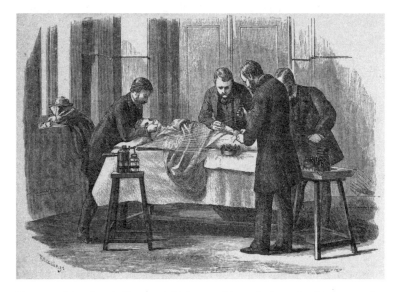

Figure 10 Lister's carbolic spray which proved how the hazards of post-operative infection could be diminished. It was eventually replaced by aseptic techniques of sterilizing instruments and the operating environment.

Rather, she wrote, 'our work begins afterward, when the poor soul comes to himself, sick, faint, and wandering; full of strange pains and confused visions, of disagreeable sensations and sights. Then we must sooth and sustain, tend and watch; preaching and practicing patience.'[172] Nursing involvement with surgery deepened with the adoption of antisepsis routines from the 1860s onwards, which created new duties of administering carbolic spray and swabbing patient and surgeon.

The Civil War also had its own 'Lady of the Lamp' in the form of Clara Barton, known as 'angel of the battlefield'. Clara travelled with military ambulances to help the sick and wounded as they were transported to the hospitals. She began a national campaign to identify 22,000 unknown soldiers after the war and in 1869 became involved with the International Red Cross (founded during the Crimean War) distributing supplies to France and Germany during the Franco-Prussian War. As in earlier wars, medical supplies including chloroform were high on the list of wants. Many surgeons volunteered to help the armies and the international Aid Society at Basle attracted many volunteers, including Russian surgeon Pirogoff. One of the first actions of the Red Cross was to take chloroform into Strasbourg after its seizure: 'probably the first instance of such mitigation of the horrors of a siege', noted William MacCormac in his *Notes and Recollections of an Ambulance Surgeon* (1871). At the end of the war, having been awarded the Iron Cross by the German emperor, Clara returned home to found the American Red Cross.

By the time of the Boer Wars anaesthesia was integral to routine military practice. Supplies of chloroform and ether were sent to each base hospital; mounted officers were given a bottle of chloroform in their saddlebag. Practical problems and scarcity of anaesthetic skills in military practitioners would continue to dog anaesthetic practice in the First World War and beyond. But the intellectual battle had been won: for severely wounded soldiers and civilians, anaesthesia was deemed to be a blessing.

6

. . . .

THE DARK SIDE
OF CHLOROFORM

Chloroform was the Jekyll and Hyde of the Victorian drug market. Its anaesthetic powers cocooned patients in oblivion, protected them from the pain and suffering of operations, and enshrined the humanitarian impulse of modern civilization. It could also serve as the antithesis of all that was good and merciful becoming, in criminal hands, a highly effective tool of manipulation and control. Its associations with abductions, murders, and rape cases, as well as its well-known predilection to kill patients who inhaled it during surgery without warning, fuelled myths and legends about its potency. Small wonder that a fear of chloroform lurked in the Victorian imagination for the rest of the nineteenth century and beyond: we may even attribute modern anxieties about the anaesthetic process to the legacy of its dark side.

Street robbers had found a 'new and most serious mode of attack', warned 'HN' in a letter to *The Times* in October 1849. His elderly relative had been seized from behind one evening whilst walking through Chester Square and became 'instantly insensible'. Coming round after 'an agreeable dream', he hazily recollected three men. His purse, keys, spectacles, and gold eyeglass were gone and his pockets ransacked: he alerted the police to the attack. Apart from a sore and swollen throat resulting from the 'ruffianly grasp', the victim recovered without incident.[173] Further reports followed. Frederick Jewett, a reputable solicitor, awoke naked in a locked bedroom in January 1850 after being mugged by Margaret Higgins and Elizabeth Smith. Smith admitted to her neighbour that she was given chloroform by her partner, Gallagher, who had stolen it from the London hospital. Higgins and Smith were sentenced to fifteen years imprisonment for the crime at the Old Bailey. Only weeks later, Charlotte Wilson was imprisoned for ten years for using a 'deleterious article such as chloroform' to rob a man walking along the Borough Road, south of the Thames towards London Bridge. One doctor reading these reports became incensed with the inaccuracy of journalistic assumptions regarding the powers of chloroform.

John Snow had penned a missive to the *London Medical Gazette* to establish the proper scientific facts surrounding chloroform. His points were clear. First, chloroform's pungency was so unique, no one could take a single breath of it without noticing; second, chloroform could only be administered by force, or with consent; and third, it did not act immediately. Given these facts, Snow suggested that any person seized on the street would hold their breath and resist the assault—their struggles would attract attention. Highly sceptical of journalists—a handkerchief 'is most likely ... the ingenious invention of the reporter'—Snow had no doubt that some shady characters 'who have to account for being in disreputable places and company' would replace previously lame excuses of 'dining out' with tales of waving handkerchiefs.[174] How Jewett found himself naked in a locked bedroom, Snow could not say, but he was adamant that neither the details of this case, nor that of the Wilson mugging, matched the profile of chloroform.

The months of 1850 passed—William Wordsworth died and Alfred Lord Tennyson became the new poet laureate; a telegraph cable was laid under the English Channel; the Swedish soprano Jenny Lind made her first tour of America—and reports of chloroform muggings continued to make headline news. In November, the *Kendal Mercury and Northern Advertiser* reported a serious attack on an elderly clergyman lodging in a temperance hotel in Kendal. On retiring for the night, the clergyman had secured his door with a chair (there was no lock) but once in bed he was attacked by a man who had hidden in the room and tried to overpower him with a chloroform-soaked towel. The clergyman struggled hard and loud; the landlord and other lodgers came to his aid. It transpired his attacker had travelled in the same stagecoach to Kendal and learnt that the clergyman was in possession of eleven gold sovereigns which he had collected for the Home Missions fund. Eighteen months imprisonment was far too lenient a sentence, wrote the editor of the *London Medical Gazette*. Snow agreed: it was a very serious case; in the dark, and without any experience of administering chloroform, the thief could have killed the clergyman by overdosage.

Chloroform's potency was heightened by its powers to tranquilize the most dangerous of wild animals. In June 1850, a hunting leopard, presented to the London Zoological Society by the Pasha of Egypt, caught one of its hind legs in the bars of its cage and in its haste to free itself, suffered a compound fracture. A sponge moistened with chloroform was tied to the end of a stick and pushed against the leopard's mouth and nose. It complained loudly, but eventually succumbed, lying quiet and motionless. Professor Simmonds of the Royal Veterinary College amputated the limb; the leopard recovered quickly, gambolling about on three legs. A year later, the grizzly bears at the London Zoo needed veterinary treatment. First secured by a collar, then held whilst chloroform was given to them, they became as docile as pussycats. Snow was swift to point out that the bears were 'entirely under control' before chloroform was given. Few picked up on such subtlety.

In Snow's view, accurate scientific facts should dissipate public fear of chloroform's powers; but politicians looked to legislation rather than science. In June 1851, Lord Campbell introduced a bill which punished unlawful use of chloroform or other stupefying drugs with a minimum of seven years imprisonment or transportation. Snow challenged the wisdom of this action: the use of force was already established as a criminal offence and could be used in cases of chloroform misuse; naming chloroform in the bill would exacerbate 'the groundless fears of the public', he told Lord Campbell.[175]

Support for Snow's views came from many quarters. *Household Words*, edited by Charles Dickens, robustly defended Snow's stance: 'it is no more easy to stupefy anyone against their will by means of chloroform, than it is by means of brandy and water,' declared the weekly magazine in May 1851.[176] But the Government held its ground and the bill was passed.

Either criminals were unperturbed by the new Act or journalists failed to take Snow's facts on board. Only months later in Manchester, a joiner was robbed by two men 'of very blackguard appearance' after being given a drink and at once becoming insensible and remaining unconscious for several hours. Chloroform must have been put in the drink, concluded the *Manchester Courier*. For a time at least, chloroform was the first consideration of police and coroners in any suspicious death. Snow had developed a method of detecting the presence of chloroform in corpses after he had been consulted about the suspicious death of a housekeeper in Clapham in 1850. He was also sent body parts to analyse after a woman had been found dead in mysterious circumstances in Wandsworth Road.

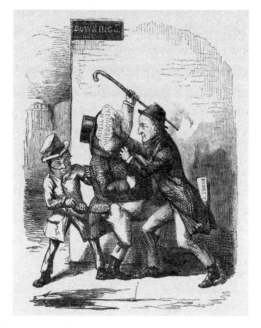

Figure 11 The new tool of criminals: aided by chloroform, thieves attempt to rob John Bull of unwelcome tax measures. *Punch* (1851).

Anxieties about the criminal use of chloroform had undoubtedly built on the fear surrounding an epidemic of poison cases during the 1840s. Reports of poison trials in *The Times* newspaper almost doubled between the 1830s and the 1840s. The poison which caused most alarm was arsenic, known as 'the murderer's choice', and estimated to be the cause of 50–75 per cent of poison deaths. Arsenic, commented the *London Medical Gazette* in 1850, was 'peculiarly adapted to the purposes of secret assassination'. A series of suspicious deaths in Essex in the late 1840s carried out by a group of local women created such public concern about the dangers of poisons that legislation was introduced to restrict open sales of arsenic. Manchester and Stockport, through local Acts of Parliament, had introduced restrictions on the sale of arsenic and prussic acid in the 1840s. In 1851 the rest of Britain followed. Chemists and other retailers were required by law to sell only to adults; maintain a register of names, addresses, and occupations of purchasers, together with date, quantity, and purpose of purchase; mix arsenic with soot or indigo so it was easily noticed; and to sell only in the presence of a witness who, with retailer and purchaser, was obliged to sign the register. The Arsenic Act won widespread support from the medical community. It also raised new concerns about the proper limits of state intervention and violation of individual liberty. The philosopher John Stuart Mill wrote his essay *On Liberty* in the wake of the Arsenic Act. How far may liberty be legitimately invaded for the prevention of crime? pondered Mill, and used the sale of poisons to analyse the principles of state responsibility versus individual freedoms. The dilemma was balancing the prevention of crime using poisons, whilst preserving the liberty of those who wished to purchase such substances for innocent domestic, manufacturing, or agricultural purposes. In the home, arsenic was a highly effective method of vermin control—although the terrible smell of mice rotting underneath floorboards was off-putting, noted *Cassell's Household Guide*. Sheep dips, fabric dyes, and a myriad of useful objects like flypapers depended on the poison. Probably, concluded Mill, the measures introduced by the Arsenic Act provided a satisfactory compromise. In chloroform's case, legislation was not sufficient to quell anxiety about its powers and fears continued.

Chloroform's ability to produce instantaneous insensibility became one of the urban myths of the nineteenth century. A 'tall man in a smock frock' visited my shop, asking for 'a liquid which occasioned insensibility with a quick smell of the bottle'—he said he had a giddiness in the head, reported a chemist to *The Times*.[177] The chemist was streetwise: he retorted 'Bosh!' and refused the sale, he declared, and explained that chloroform did not have the chemical capabilities to act instantaneously; an ammonia-based compound was far more promising. Inaccuracies persisted and so did muggings. In 1857 whilst walking on a country road, Mrs Elizabeth Savage, a housekeeper, was overpowered by highwaymen, supposedly with chloroform. On regaining consciousness she found herself naked in a wood: it was some time before she gained the help of passing women. Whatever the agent used, it was a grim ordeal. In 1865 the *Lancet* lambasted misrepresentations of chloroform in the popular press. Such journals 'have no doubt about the fact that a highwayman can, by shaking a handkerchief impregnated with chloroform under the nose of his victim, produce instantaneous insensibility'.[178] But the *Lancet's* invective, like Snow's protestations, failed to reassert the facts about chloroform in the public domain. Chloroform's grip on the Victorian imagination was buoyed up by the literature of the day.

Dickens' editorial in *Household Words* may have paid homage to Snow's scientific facts surrounding chloroform. But fiction freed Dickens to employ the popular myths surrounding chloroform's potency and its use in muggings. *A Tale of Two Cities*, published in instalments in 1859, and set in London and Paris, drew much from Thomas Carlyle's *A History of the French Revolution*. French aristocrat Darnay and English barrister Carton are both in love with Lucie Manette but Carton performs the ultimate sacrifice by taking Darnay's place at the guillotine and setting him free for Lucie. Chloroform is not mentioned by name, but its hallmarks are unmistakable. Carton enters a 'small, dim, crooked' chemist's shop kept by a 'small, dim, crooked man', passes a slip of paper across the counter that causes the chemist to whistle softly and caution, 'you will be careful to keep them separate … you know the consequences of mixing them?' before passing Carton some small packets. Visiting

Darnay the next day, Carton persuades him to exchange clothes and pen a final letter. Carton moves his hand slowly and softly close to Darnay's face: 'What vapour is that?', Darnay asks. Within a few minutes his pen trails off into 'unintelligible signs'; soon his body was 'stretched insensible' on the ground. After Darnay is born away to safety, Carton faces the guillotine, secure in the knowledge that 'It is a far, far better thing that I do, than I have ever done'. For other writers too, chloroform became an indispensable literary device. Arthur Conan Doyle used chloroform in several Sherlock Holmes stories. Mrs Maberley was chloroformed by intruders in 'The Three Gables' and her account chimed with reports of chloroform muggings: 'I was conscious for a moment of the chloroform rag which was thrust over my mouth, but I have no notion how long I may have been senseless. When I woke, one man was at the bedside and another was rising with a bundle in his hand,' Mrs Maberley, looking pale and ill, told Holmes and Watson.

Chloroform also became a popular self-help remedy for a spectrum of aches and pains: asthma, headache, toothache, and sleeplessness were but a few of the ailments which could be relieved by breathing a few drops on a hanky. Though poorly soluble in water, mixing the chemical with oil, fat, or soda water extended its uses: injected into the rectum or the vagina it could relieve local irritability and pain. Doctors may have counselled against its use but chloroform was freely available. In 1855 the British Indian Army doctor J. Collis Browne created chlorodyne—a preparation containing chloroform, cannabis, opium, and peppermint. It became one of the most popular patent remedies of the nineteenth century. Chlorodyne 'relieves pain, calms the system, restores the damaged functions ... Old and Young may take it at all hours', proclaimed advertisements. Thousands of Victorians bought chlorodyne; versions of the preparation were sold until recently. But chlorodyne was addictive and deaths from overdosage were common, as were deaths from the self-administration of chloroform.

In June 1850, young Mr Smith, staying at his friend Mr Ray's house, was heard to moan during the night. In the morning he was found dead in bed, a handkerchief pressed to his mouth and nostrils. Smith inhaled chloroform to relieve face-ache; he knew it was risky—he often asked William Girt, groom to Mr Ray, to sit with him and rouse him when he became insensible. The coroner at the inquest offered his deepest sympathy to Smith's relatives: his own nephew, Walter Badger, had died from chloroform during a tooth extraction. Nor was specialist knowledge of chloroform proof against its dangers. John Roberts, manager of a chemist's shop, was found dead in bed with a silk handkerchief in his hand and an empty phial of chloroform. He used chloroform to deaden pains in his face. Even when self-administration of chloroform had medical approval the process was fraught with danger. The death of Mrs Childers, 'one of [society's] happiest ornaments', was the subject of a letter to *The Times* in December 1875 by her doctor, Robert Ellis. Author of a book entitled *The Safe Abolition of Pain*, Ellis was, perhaps, concerned as much to protect his reputation as to contribute to the debate surrounding chloroform's risks and benefits. Mrs Childers used very small measured doses of chloroform to relieve pain and obtain sleep: Ellis explained how she measured out between 10 and 20 minims into a small phial in order to ensure complete safety. When she was discovered, the little phial was by her side, but her hand was grasping the large bottle of chloroform and its glass stopper was on the floor. Ellis replaced the stopper and found that in a few minutes of being held in a warm hand, the remaining fluid inside the bottle expanded in the warmth and forced the stopper out. It was an accident waiting to happen. Ellis painted a picture of Mrs Childers inhaling from the small phial whilst continuing to hold the bottle of chloroform. As she relaxed and became drowsy, the warmth of her hand caused the pressure to build inside the chloroform bottle until the stopper flew out: 'from that fatal moment her death was sealed. The pillow, bedclothes, and nightdress became quite soaked with the fluid, and the narcotism, deepening with every inspiration, terminated in a death as peaceful as sleep.'[179] How could such an accident have been avoided?, Ellis ruminated. To lessen chloroform's risks in general anaesthesia, Ellis customarily mixed it with ether. But ladies making social visits would not tolerate ether's pungency on their breath, he explained pragmatically.

Anaesthetic agents were all potentially addictive—Humphry Davy had swiftly realized nitrous oxide's addictive qualities and ether claimed addicts. One of the earliest deaths caused by chloroform addiction was that of an Aberdeen chemist's assistant 17-year-old Arthur Walker. He adored the exhilaration and excitement of chloroform—he habitually inhaled it from his handkerchief. Arthur's father was foreman at the same chemist's and forbid him access to chloroform. But one day Arthur was left alone with a younger assistant: he could not resist the lure of chloroform and became very excited, staggering about the shop all morning. Then he laid a towel on the serving counter, poured on chloroform, and placed his face on it. The young assistant was scared to approach: he knew Arthur could be violent after chloroform inhaling. But when he did venture forwards Arthur was lifeless. Doctors were called, resuscitation was attempted by making a hole in his windpipe, and the lungs were inflated for more than an hour. But chloroform had taken Arthur beyond oblivion.

Addiction and drug dependency cast a slur in Victorian society—reports of Arthur Walker's death stressed that suffocation, rather than addiction, was the cause of death. Family and friends were anxious to avoid victims being labelled as addicts, especially respectable middle-class ladies like Lucy Elwes of Whitby. About to have a child, Lucy was found dead by her doctor who had been staying over in case labour came on. Family and servants tried to hide the truth, but it was eventually revealed that Lucy often used chloroform to soothe toothache during the night. Another victim of 'the powerful and insidious soporific' was the wife of the Revd Alexander Gregory from Anstruther, near Dundee, who was found dead in bed in the morning with a handkerchief over her mouth. Feeling unwell like Lucy, Mrs Gregory resorted to inhaling chloroform to bring sleep. Occasionally addiction gave cause for pride. At the inquest of a 42-two-year-old midwife in 1888, relatives boasted that her habit of inhaling a pint of chloroform a day fitted her to be the world champion chloroform taker.

The appearance of chloroform at the heart of one of the most notorious murder trials of the 1800s—the Pimlico Mystery—cemented it in the public's imagination as a dangerous and potent chemical. *The Penny Illustrated Paper* described how, on 12 April 1886, Adelaide Bartlett with a 'great shock of short black hair', a 'broad and sallow face', and stupefied by pain or grief stood before Mr Justice Wills at the Old Bailey, accused of the murder of her husband, Thomas Edwin Bartlett, on 1 January of that year. Also charged as an accessory to the fact was the Revd George Dyson, a 28-year-old Methodist minister who played third party in the curious *ménage à trois* (although charges against Dyson were dropped at the commencement of proceedings). The trial was a London sensation. Crowds packed the courtroom; ladies took the best seats—'How is it that women will crowd a criminal court to see another of their sex in such a painful position?', mused the *Pall Mall Gazette* in one of its daily instalments of the trial which were read avidly by those unable to witness first hand the extraordinary unfolding of the Bartlett's Victorian melodrama.

The Bartletts had met in 1874 when Adelaide was around 16 years of age. Her origins were dubious; her paternity was never confirmed. Edwin was a grocer, animated by the laws of supply and demand, and the minutiae of trade; his father took against Adelaide from the start. Living with Edwin's father and brothers created tensions; there were suggestions that Adelaide had tried to run away with Fred, Edwin's younger brother. Some years after the marriage Adelaide gave birth to a stillborn child; she had taken advice from Mary Gove Nichols, who promoted natural childbirth rather than easing labour pains with chloroform. By 1884 the Bartletts had moved to a cottage in the village of Merton Abbey, near Wimbledon where Edwin had space to indulge his interest: the breeding of St Bernard dogs. Here enters the Revd George Dyson and here begins their extraordinary *ménage à trois*.

Appointed to the local Methodist chapel, Dyson became friends with the Bartletts. Dyson taught, walked with, and lunched with Adelaide: 'my husband threw us together. He requested us to kiss in his presence and he seemed to enjoy it,' she later said. The mutual dependency was clear in 1885 when Dyson took up a post in Putney; the Bartletts moved to Pimlico, taking rooms on the first floor of 85 Claverdon Street, home of Frederick Doggett, a registrar of births, marriages, and deaths and his wife, Caroline. Edwin continued in the grocery trade, spending each day tasting around 300 samples of tea, cheese, and butter from his chain of 6 shops in south London. His annual income was around £300, a good middle-class living, particularly as he had no children to support. Always in good health, Edwin had obtained a life insurance of £400 from the British Equitable Life Association after passing a physical examination. But within a few months of arriving in Pimlico, Edwin had a severe attack of vomiting, diarrhoea, and stomach cramps. A local doctor, Dr Alfred Leach, was called to the house and on examination spotted 'a deep bluish-red margin' along Edwin's gums. Leach immediately recognized it as a classic mark of mercury poisoning. Mercury was a popular treatment for venereal disease; Leach assumed Edwin had syphilis. But Edwin denied this, and an examination of the genital area ruled this out. Leach later summarized the possibilities: had Edwin been practising suicidal experiments? Was he a victim of a poisoner? Or had he simply had a very strong reaction to a single dose of mercury? Edwin's explanation was that he had taken a blue pill of unknown origin from a drawer of old samples in a grocer's shop; Leach assumed that this must have contained some element of mercury. It is reasonable to guess that Edwin took this pill in an attempt to relieve toothache.

Despite his robust physical health, Edwin's teeth left everything to be desired. He could not bear to have his teeth or gums touched by his own or another person's finger, nor indeed by a toothbrush. In the 1870s most of Edwin's teeth were sawn down to gum level and replaced with an artificial set. That it was very difficult to achieve a good fit of artificial teeth without removing the roots was well known. Indeed it was one of the problems that occupied American dentists like Horace Wells and William Morton in the 1840s and led to experiments with nitrous oxide and ether. Edwin's artificial teeth hurt his mouth so much he obtained another set but the pain was so great he discarded them. He also abandoned cleaning his teeth. Offensive breath and rotten teeth were the first things Leach noticed about Edwin when he met him in 1885. Edwin had not capitalized on anaesthesia to relieve the pain of having roots extracted: 'laughing gas' did not work on him, he told Leach. Previous attempts to inhale nitrous oxide during dentistry had failed: the doctors and dentists supervising his case told him he 'could never be brought under'. Leach resorted to hypnotizing Edwin while some of his rotten teeth were removed and it seemed to break the spell. On 31

December 1885, the day before Edwin died, one of his canine teeth was removed under nitrous oxide, although he had to breathe a great deal of the gas and recovered exceptionally rapidly. He was on the road to recovery, thought Leach. Highly relieved by the success of the extraction, Edwin returned home where he ate a good supper and ordered extra breakfast for the following morning a good piece of haddock would encourage him to rise early, he said. Landlady Caroline Doggett visited her tenants during the evening: out of the blue, Adelaide asked her if she had had experience of chloroform; Caroline said, yes, she had inhaled it for an operation some years ago. Adelaide did not mention her own supply of chloroform purchased on her behalf by Dyson. She had told Dyson she needed chloroform to soothe Edwin: Dyson visited three separate chemists in Putney and Wimbledon under the pretext of needing the chemical to remove stains to gain the quantities Adelaide requested. What happened in the hours following remains a mystery to this day.

Since Edwin's illness Adelaide had sat with him through the night; he would only sleep if she held his foot. 'A kinder, more tender, more patient, or more self-sacrificing nurse could not have been wished for,' remembered Leach, perhaps as besotted with her as Dyson had been.[180] But at some point during the early hours of 1 January 1886, Edwin had swallowed chloroform. Adelaide told of waking and finding Edwin dead, of trying to revive him with brandy, sending for Leach, and waking the Doggetts. For Adelaide it was unfortunate, perhaps, that her landlord was familiar with the rules governing suspicious deaths. On entering the room, Frederick Doggett noticed a pungent smell coming from a brandy glass on the mantelpiece: he refused to register the death until a post-mortem had been carried out. Edwin's father was sent for—his dislike of Adelaide had persisted through the marriage—he accused her of killing his son. The post-mortem revealed that Edwin died from chloroform poisoning: chloroform was found in his stomach contents. The Home Office analyst Dr Thomas Stevenson noted in his casebook,

> I cannot say exactly how much chloroform had been taken ... I am of the opinion that the appearances in the stomach, coupled with the quantity of chloroform found in the contents of the stomach, and also its presence in the fluid from the intestines point to the administration of a fatal dose of chloroform, in the liquid form, by the mouth.[181]

How chloroform had been administered, Stevenson could not explain. Adelaide's response was extraordinary. She confided to Leach the unsavoury details of her marriage: no sexual relationship with her husband; Edwin's fostering of the relationship between her and Dyson and his giving of her to Dyson as a future wife after his own demise. But then, she said, Edwin had attempted to renew sexual intimacy: she could not tolerate this because of her commitment to Dyson. (Edwin's rotten teeth could not have aided his suit.) She planned to wave a chloroformed hanky in front of Edwin's face to encourage sleep rather than lust although she had later regretted her intentions, confessed, and given Edwin the bottle of chloroform. She claimed the bottle was present on the mantelpiece when Doggett entered the room; it was assumed that it had been thrown away in error for it was never found.

Adelaide was not allowed to testify in her own defence when the case came to trial. (Only in 1898 did the Criminal Evidence Act give the accused the right to testify.) Her barrister was Edward Clarke, later famous for his defence of Oscar Wilde in the Queensbury case. Clarke's eloquent presentation to the jury portrayed Adelaide as a devoted wife and nurse, a model of feminine virtues. But the trial revealed titillating details about the strange sexual relationship between Adelaide and Edwin. A book on birth control found in the house was morally dangerous, cautioned Judge Wills—reading this 'helped to unsex' the couple, he added. According to Adelaide, 'the more attention and admiration I gained from ... male acquaintances the more delighted did he [Edwin] appear. Their attention to me gave him pleasure.' Clarke implied Edwin was the driver of the sexual peculiarities in the relationship—Edwin's father admitted that his son believed it would be best to have two wives: 'one to take out and one to do the work'.[182] The prosecution, led by Attorney General Sir Charles Russell QC, argued that Adelaide made Edwin insensible with chloroform whilst he was asleep then poured it down his throat. But Clarke produced firm evidence which showed how difficult it was to use chloroform successfully on sleeping adults, let alone judge the precise degree of anaesthesia in which the swallowing reflex remained. And Stevenson's evidence that he had found no burn or other trace of chloroform in Bartlett's mouth or oesophagus confirmed that it must have been administered whilst Bartlett was both upright and able to swallow. A host of theories abounded. Clarke believed Edwin had committed suicide on account of his mental depression: he stressed that chloroform had no precedent as an agent of murder. The *Lancet* pointed out that though the method of administering chloroform could not be proved, this alone was no reason not to charge Adelaide with murder. It cited the case of William Palmer, convicted and hanged in 1856 for the murder of his associate, John Cook, by strychnine, even though strychnine had not been found in Cook's body. Leach, clearly under Adelaide's spell, vouched that Edwin attempted to spite Adelaide after her revelations by taking some chloroform, but accidentally overdosed himself. Was Adelaide a devoted wife, an 'angel of the house', or a manipulative poisoner and murderess? The jury was gravely suspicious of Adelaide but could not convict because of lack of evidence. After the trial, a letter from the foreman to a newspaper revealed how the majority of jurors believed Edwin to have committed suicide, either deliberately or inadvertently. The public supported her acquittal. The roar of cheering that burst from onlookers in- and outside the court provoked Judge Wills to bellow, 'This conduct is an outrage. A court of justice is not to be turned into a theatre.'[183] Doctors remained perplexed: 'Now that it is all over, she should tell us, in the interest of science, how she did it,' commented Sir James Paget, surgeon at St Bartholomew's hospital. But she never did. The question of how chloroform got into Edwin's stomach has remained hanging since 1886, though the case has stimulated film makers and writers, most depicting Adelaide as the villainess.

Chloroform enabled criminal activities. It also became a weapon in the hands of unscrupulous doctors. From the beginning, concerns had been raised about the dangers arising from unconsciousness, particularly for female patients who became insensible, not just to pain, but to any form of abuse that may be perpetrated by the medical practitioner.

'A new crime', pronounced *The Times* in November 1847, telling of a French dentist who had been found guilty of assaulting two young women—Hyacinthe and Henriette—whilst they were under the influence of ether. Hyacinthe reported that she was aware of what Laine was doing but was 'totally unable to offer any resistance'. Ether's effects on the imagination had caused the women to take their 'hallucinations for facts', argued Laine's advocate. But evidence of agitation and dishevelment of clothes convinced the jury of Laine's guilt. He was sentenced to six years hard labour and ordered to pay damages. 'You have condemned an innocent man! It was to obtain money that Mademoiselle Hyacinthe prosecuted me!', vehemently declaimed Laine as he was led away.[184] It was a protest that would be repeated in different forms over the next decades, particularly as chloroform was so much easier to breathe.

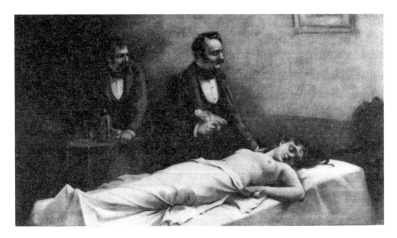

Figure 12 This picture emphasises the vulnerability of the female patient under anaesthesia as the doctors survey her naked body with, perhaps, more than medical interest, 1896.

In retrospect, some cases of chloroform abuse appear clear-cut yet perpetrators escaped for lack of definitive evidence. In a bid to have her virtue verified, 24-year-old Lucy Ashby was taken by her father to be examined by Richard Freeman, a surgeon in Deptford in 1870. Her mother accused Lucy of sexual intimacy with a young man during the Easter Monday festivities. Freeman asked her father to wait outside whilst he examined her. Lucy told how Freeman asked her to smell a bottle of liquid then shake it; the liquid splashed and burnt her skin—and then stupefied her. Opening her eyes, Lucy saw Freeman holding an instrument in his hand. When her father entered the room, Freeman confirmed Lucy's virginity was intact, but Lucy complained of assault. Her father took her to Dr David Hope, who confirmed evidence of assault: Lucy's description of the apple taste of the liquid suggested the agent was chloroform, said Hope. Freeman went to trial and was found not guilty although the judge warned him never to examine a patient without a witness present. This was not the first time Freeman had slid through the net of justice. Three years earlier, then practising as a dentist, Freeman had been accused of raping a young woman whilst she was under the influence of chloroform. The balance of evidence was not thought to be in the young woman's favour. Freeman had escaped, only to commit a similar crime some years later.

In Lucy's case, the instrument of abuse was most probably the speculum which entered gynaecological practice in the 1840s amidst protests about its propensity to promote immorality. Introduced in France by physician Joseph Recamier, the speculum was used by Paris police to examine prostitutes for venereal disease. British doctors like William Acton, best known for his work on genital–urinary diseases and prostitution, and William Jones, founder of the Samaritan Free Hospital for Women, argued that the speculum facilitated correct diagnosis: vaginal discharge was a symptom found in a whole range of diseases. But the instrument was 'unjustifiable on the grounds of propriety and morality', countered Robert Lee, Professor of Midwifery at St George's Hospital; it was absolutely the last resort for diagnosis. Again the debate hinged on the complex inter-relations of female sexuality and morality: 'the female who has been subjected to such treatment is not the same person in delicacy and purity as she was before,' explained Marshall Hall. The speculum dulled the 'edge of virgin modesty' and sullied the 'pure minds of the daughters of England'. As had been the case with ether, doctors expressed a fear that the speculum could unleash female sexuality until it became ungovernable. Robert Brudenell Carter in his 1853 study of hysteria cautioned,

> I have, more than once, seen young unmarried women, of the middle classes of society, reduced, by the constant use of the speculum, to the mental and moral condition of prostitutes; seeking to give themselves the same indulgence by the practice of solitary vice; and asking

THE DARK SIDE OF CHLOROFORM

every medical practitioner, under whose care they fell, to institute an examination of the sexual organs.[185]

In the end, disputes over the moral questions raised by the speculum were solved by anaesthesia; unconsciousness shrouded female sensibilities from its dangers. By the 1880s patients at the Chelsea Hospital for Women in London were routinely given chloroform before speculum examinations.

One of the most bizarre instances of rape under chloroform claims was the 1864 trial of Travers *v*. Wilde. Sir William Wilde, father of Oscar, specialized in the eye and the ear. He established St Mark's Hospital in Dublin in 1844, wrote textbooks, collected the first statistics on deafness, blindness, and eye and ear diseases in Ireland, and was Surgeon Oculist to the Queen in Ireland. He also had a penchant for pretty girls: he fathered three illegitimate children before his marriage to Jane Elgee in 1851. The Wildes were a striking pair, not just physically—he was of average stature, she was nearly 6 foot tall—but in their talent for holding vivacious receptions for an eclectic mix of actors, musicians, politicians, and university professors. Wilde used chloroform in his practice: he had corresponded with its discoverer, James Simpson, on various medical matters including leprosy and puerperal fever. In 1854 Wilde took on a new patient, 18-year-old Mary Travers: 'a nice-looking woman, of pleasing voice and intelligent countenance.' According to Mary, in October 1862 Wilde gave her chloroform in his consulting room and then raped her. Mary said nothing until 1864 when, prompted by jealousy perhaps of the public admiration enjoyed by the Wildes— he received his knighthood in January 1864; she had been highly praised for her translation of *The First Temptation* by M. Schwab in 1863—Mary wrote threatening letters to the press and published a pamphlet about Dr and Mrs Quilp—the Wildes—under the name

140

of Speranza (the pen name of Jane Wilde). The pamphlet described an abortive attempt by Dr Quilp, under the 'instrumentality of chloroform', to destroy a young girl's virtue. Mary gave copies of the pamphlet to the Wildes' servants. Jane Wilde complained directly to Mary's father, Professor of Medical Jurisprudence at Trinity College, Dublin, about these 'unfounded' accusations. Professor Travers replied, saying he knew of no reason why Mary should pursue such a course of action. All may have resolved itself but Mary discovered Jane's letter to her father and sued her for libel. Chloroform, it turned out, had not featured in the case. Rather, Mary admitted in court that she settled upon chloroform because it had such a 'treacherous' reputation. On cross-examination, Mary conceded that she had continued to visit Wilde for medical care after the rape. She also accepted presents and borrowed money; he had given her money for her fare to Australia but she had not left the country. The trial lasted five days in December 1864 and the jury finally upheld the charge of libel though the award of damages of one farthing to Mary suggested questions hung over her innocence. Wilde had to pay Jane's costs of £2,000. Though several letters of Wilde's to Mary, produced at the trial, indicated he was not without fault, his reputation did not suffer: 'all Dublin has called on us to offer their sympathy, and all the medical profession here and in London have sent letters to express their entire disbelief of the (in fact) impossible charge,' wrote Jane to her Swedish friend Rosalie Olivecrona.[186] Her optimism was reflected by the *Lancet* editorial: 'Sir William Wilde will have no want of sympathisers. Such is the natural reward of a life devoted to scientific research, of a free heart, and of a generous hand.'[187] Nevertheless, the case became immortalized in a student ditty:

> An eminent oculist lives in the Square,
> His skill is unrivalled, his talent is rare,

And if you will listen I'll certainly try
To tell how he opened Miss Travers's eye.[188]

It also presaged his son, Oscar's own trial some thirty years later. The aphrodisiacal effects of anaesthetics had caused alarm since 1846. Then, excitement particularly in female patients was explained through moralistic shortcomings. By the 1880s physiology was used to rationalize female behaviour: 'Chloroform, ether, nitrous oxide, gas, cocaine ... possess the property of exciting sexual emotions, and in many cases produce erotic hallucinations. It is undoubted that in certain persons sexual orgasm may occur during the induction of anaesthesia,' explained Dudley Wilmot Buxton, anaesthetist at University College Hospital in *Anaesthetics, Their Uses and Adminis-tration*, published in 1888. There were undoubtedly 'designing, bad women'—Mary Travers possibly—who falsely accused doctors of abuse under chloroform, said Buxton, but it was also possible for 'modest, virtuous and refined gentlewomen' to hallucinate and then claim violation.[189] Chaperonage of anaesthesia was essential if such charges were to be avoided, advised Buxton. Birmingham surgeon George Howard, accused of the rape of Fanny Child in 1877, had been released after a posse of medical men gave evidence of the oc-currence of sexual hallucinations under anaesthesia. Benjamin Ward Richardson, friend of John Snow, described how a young lady had made precisely the same charge as Fanny Child against her dentist. Fortunately for the dentist, her father and mother and two doc-tors were present. Medical anxieties persist. The introduction of the anaesthetic propofol in the 1980s caused some patients to display amorous, disinhibited behaviour: 'I agree strongly ... that a third party should be present ... in view of the possibility of laying oneself open to allegations of sexual impropriety,' wrote one Manchester anaesthetist.[190]

Prostitution had a long history in Britain but from the 1860s Josephine Butler headed a campaign against the Contagious Diseases Acts (1864, 1868, and 1869) under which any woman found in the street could be apprehended and taken for a medical examination regardless of any evidence of prostitution. Butler drew attention to the inequities inherent in the legislation: males visiting prostitutes were depicted as fulfilling a 'natural impulse', whereas the women were cast as wicked and immoral. Butler also uncovered the scandal of young British girls being abducted and taken to work in European brothels. In 1885 startling revelations in the *Pall Mall Gazette* raised the debate to new levels. Chloroform was again at the heart of the matter.

Prostitution, said William Thomas Stead, editor of the *Pall Mall Gazette*, was 'the ghastliest curse which haunts civilized society'. But his interest in sexuality fell little short of an obsession: 'His repressed sexuality was, I consider, the motive force of many of his activities,' said his friend Henry Havelock Ellis, whose radical work on sexual psychology shaped twentieth-century understandings.[191] Stead's intention was to raise the age of consent from 13 to 16 years old: a bill was supposedly in preparation but politicians seemed half-hearted. Stead's jaded confidence in state mechanisms prompted him to initiate a piece of investigative journalism that blurred to a greater extent than ever before the boundaries between reporting and creating news. The first article in a four-part saga entitled 'The Maiden Tribute of Modern Babylon' was published on 6 July 1885. Stead's intention was to provide proof of the dark and seamy underworld of Victorian vice and prostitution, and specifically of the sale, purchase, and violation of children; the procuration of virgins; entrapping and ruin of women; and the international slave trade in girls. These facts were common knowledge. Stead's view was that definitive evidence might stimulate action. Helped by Mrs Rebecca

Jarrett, a reformed ex-prostitute working for the Salvation Army, Stead set up a complicated chain of events: the purchase of a young girl; confirmation of her virginity; proof that in the right circumstances this could be sullied. Jarrett procured Eliza Armstrong, 13-year-old daughter of a chimney-sweep and Eliza's mother was paid £5 in recompense for her daughter. Jarrett later claimed she had made it plain to Mrs Armstrong that Eliza's future lay in vice, not domesticity. Eliza's virginity was proved by Mme Louise Mourez, a known abortionist. Here chloroform enters the story. Mourez sold a bottle of chloroform to Sampson Jacques, the colleague of Stead who had accompanied Jarrett and Eliza for the examination. He took Eliza and Jarrett to a brothel in Poland Street: Jarrett tried to persuade Eliza to breathe chloroform to get her to go to sleep quickly but failed. Stead, believing Eliza to be sleeping, entered the room. His intention was to prove how easily virtue could be sullied. But Eliza shouted out as Stead entered. Jarrett then took Eliza away from the brothel to a nursing home, where, as she lay sleeping later that night, the well-known gynaecologist Dr Heywood Smith put her under the influence of chloroform to examine her and confirm her virginity. Eliza was then sent to France to take up employment although she returned after her mother, having read the press reports, instigated her she return and took proceedings against Stead and his accomplices. At the trial, Stead was found guilty and sentenced to three months imprisonment because Eliza had been taken without her father's consent, and without written evidence regarding payment to her mother.

Public outrage against the evidence of prostitution and vice on the streets of London revealed by Stead's reports was unprecedented. Crowds mobbed the *Gazette*'s offices in Northumberland Street: the print run was extended from 8,000 to 12,000 copies—eventually the presses could cope with no more. The Salvation Army obtained nearly 4,000 signatures on a petition requesting parliamentary action on the age of consent. Its delivery to the House of Commons was an incredible public spectacle: crowds lined the route through Hackney, Shoreditch, and Bishopsgate to watch the petition—almost two and a half miles long—drawn by a wagon and followed by hundreds of marching Salvation Army soldiers. And on 14 August 1885, the age of consent was raised to 16 years of age. But Stead's manipulation of events and the inconsistencies in some of his evidence left a bitter taste for some: 'nobody ever trusted him after the discovery that the case of Eliza ... was a put-up job ... Stead deserved [imprisonment] for such a betrayal of our confidence in him,' noted George Bernard Shaw.[192] Stead maintained that the change of law stood as 'one of the greatest achievements which any journalist single-handed had ever accomplished'. He left the *Gazette* and in 1912 died on the sinking *Titanic*, sacrificing his space on the lifeboat to women and children.

The use of chloroform to supposedly dope Eliza and then perform a physical examination without her consent sparked intense criticism in the medical press. The *Lancet* railed,

It does not seem to have been made sufficiently clear at this miserable trial that only under circumstances which necessitate anaesthesia for a remedial purpose is it justifiable to administer chloroform. A certain amount of peril to life always attends the use of chloroform. ... What was the purpose of placing this girl under chloroform, thereby exposing her to peril of her life? Simply and solely that she might be examined with a view to the whitewashing of a man who had wilfully placed himself in a position to be suspected, perhaps accused, of violating her. So revolting are these details of what cannot ... be considered otherwise than as an indecent assault committed by DR HEYWOOD SMITH on ELIZA ARMSTRONG.[193]

Heywood Smith's career was reduced to tatters: he lost his position at the British Lying-In hospital; he had to resign as secretary of the British Gynaecological Society, a position he had held in recognition of his status and popularity within the specialty; and he was severely censured by the Royal College of Physicians. Heywood Smith's attempt to explain his use of chloroform as a means of protecting Eliza's moral virtue fell on stony ground.

Chloroform's power to assist the dark arts of the criminal combined with continuing surgical fatalities to create persistent patient fear of anaesthesia. Alarmingly, fear itself could trigger a fatality: 'Experience … shows that fatal results have often followed the administration of Chloroform to the persons who have exhibited decisive and unaccountable dread of it. This is a curious fact that we may account for … by some theory or instinct or some superstition of the forecast shadow of approaching fate,' remarked Charles Dickens, writing as editor of *Household Words* in 1853.[194] Few patients refused anesthesia but in 1896 'the majority of patients regard the anaesthetic with far greater dread than the operation', noted the surgeon Frederick Treves, best known for his rescue of Joseph Merrick, the 'Elephant Man', whose appalling deformities had made him a freak.[195] In the same year H. G. Wells published his short story *Under the Knife*, which captured the anxieties of patients facing an operation. 'What if I die under it? The thought recurred again and again, as I walked home … Was this dullness of feeling in itself an anticipation? … Did a man near to death begin instinctively to withdraw himself from the meshes of matter and sense,' worried Wells's protagonist. He did not die but he did experience awareness and an out-of-body experience. Chloroform was given and he 'fell motionless, and a great silence, a monstrous silence, and an impenetrable blackness came upon him.' But then awareness struck and not only could he see the operation, he could see the thoughts of surgeon Haddon and anaesthetist Mowbray. He looked into Haddon's mind

> and saw he was afraid of cutting a branch of the portal vein ... he was growing more and more nervous in his work ... his dread of cutting too little was battling with his dread of cutting too far ... a great uprush of horrible realisation set all his thoughts swirling and simultaneously I perceived that the vein was cut ... For one brief terrible moment sensation came back to me. That feeling of falling headlong which comes in nightmares, that feeling a thousand times intensified, that and a black horror swept across my thoughts in a torrent. Then ... I was in mid-air. ... whirling away through space, held to the earth by gravitation, partaking of the earth-inertia, moving in its wreath of epicycles round the sun, and with the sun and the planets on their vast march through space.

As consciousness returned 'an almost intolerable gladness and radiance rushed in upon me ... at my side I felt a subdued feeling that could scarcely be spoken of as pain. The operation had not killed me.' Few patients could claim such a dramatic experience: most would have understood the wash of relief at the restoration of consciousness.

7

· · · ·

CHANGED UNDERSTANDINGS
OF PAIN

On the morning of 26 May 1868, Michael Barrett, legs and arms
secured by leather straps, mounted the steps up to the scaf-
fold at Newgate Prison, accompanied by his priest. The hangman,
William Calcraft, put a cap over his face and a rope round his neck:
the bolt was drawn and the drop fell with a resounding boom; a great
cry rose from the crowd. 'Barrett died without a struggle,' reported
The Times. Some spectators dispersed, others remained until Calcraft
cut down Bartlett's body 'amid such a storm of yells and execrations
as has seldom been heard even from such a crowd'.[196] (Calcraft was
noted by Charles Dickens for his 'unseemly briskness, in his jokes, his
oaths, and his brandy'.) Death was certified by the prison surgeon and
Barrett was buried that evening in an unmarked grave within Newgate
prison grounds. Barrett was the five hundred and forty-fourth public
hanging at Newgate since January 1800: he was also the last. Three
days later, Parliament passed the Capital Punishment Amendment
Act (first advocated in 1813), which decreed that hangings should take
place inside prison walls. Although witnesses, including the family of
victims, would be admitted, hangings would cease to be the public
spectacle they had been since the fifth century when they were introduced as a method of execution in Anglo-Saxon Britain.

Barrett's story is well known within the history of Irish nationalism. He had been sentenced to death for his part in the bombing of Clerkenwell Prison on 13 December 1867. A member of the reactionary Irish group, the Fenians, Barrett allegedly intended to blast a hole in the prison wall and allow the escape of a Fenian prisoner, Richard O'Sullivan-Burke. But as well as demolishing the prison wall, the explosion tore through a row of houses killing twelve people, and injuring over fifty more. Only hours before the explosion, Prime Minister Benjamin Disraeli had banned Fenian meetings; the Leader of the Opposition, William Ewart Gladstone, later to become Liberal Prime Minister, began to consider the option of Home Rule. Barrett's conviction was highly contested. In 1903 when Newgate Prison was demolished, his remains were moved to the City of London Cemetery and the grave marked with a small plaque; it still attracts visits from those interested in Irish history.

Barrett's public hanging is also of high significance in the history of anaesthesia: it marks a great watershed in cultural attitudes to pain. By decisively disproving the value of pain in operations, anaesthesia had created powerful waves that spread beyond surgery and stimulated doctors to intensify their efforts to palliate the pain of chronic and terminal disease. More broadly, it sustained the growing social antipathy to pain which had emerged in the eighteenth century, and which led to profound transformations in many areas of Victorian culture. The 1870s anti-vivisection movement; the reform of the penal system from the 1860s onwards; and the reworking of pain in Christian doctrine in the 1860s may seem a diverse collection of topics. But each of these controversies was driven in large part by the new understandings of pain, which viewed its infliction, not just as inhumane, but as a great moral danger.

Prolonging life and alleviating pain were secondary only to the cure or prevention of disease, proclaimed C. J. B. Williams, physician at the Brompton Hospital for Consumption in his 1862 Lumleian lecture. Terminally ill patients show intense gratitude for 'the minor triumph of prolonging life and relieving pain', and diagnoses, even for the terminally ill, must be patient-palatable, Williams reminded his audience at the Royal College of Physicians. His concern was the effect on the patient of a diagnosis which alarmed rather than reassured. Telling patients that 'the prospect of danger' is a long way off and the pain of any disease will be alleviated produces better outcomes than fuelling anxiety by stressing their diseased condition, he argued.[197] Pain featured in many medical writings. It was 'emphatically the Nemesis by which man is pursued from the cradle to the grave', stated physician William Dale in a series of articles published in the *Lancet* in 1871. Quoting Milton's famous lines 'Pain is perfect misery, the worst of evils' and Burn's searing condemnation:

> My curse upon your venom'd stand,
> That shoots my tortured gums slang,
> And thro' my lugs gies mony a twang
> Wi' gnawing vengeance;
> Tearing my nerves wi' bitter pan, like racking engines.

Dale analysed several diseases specifically in relation to the pain they caused during their terminal stages. Tuberculosis, the largest single recorded cause of death in Britain in the nineteenth century with around one in every forty adults between the ages of twenty and sixty a sufferer at any time, was described by Charles Dickens in *Nicholas Nickleby* (1836) as 'a disease in which life and death are so strangely blended that death takes the glow and hue of life, and life the gaunt and grisly form of death'. 'Clever word-painting', remarked Dale, but it fell short of capturing the miserable end of TB victims with tubercular abscesses who experienced constant feelings of suffocation during the last stages of the disease. Cancer was the disease that caused most pain, often of a 'lancinating, neuralgic character'. (Neuralgia was thought to be a disease of the nerves, particularly those in the head, face, and uterus. Its pain was intense, like an electric shock, said Dale.) The severe and constant pain of cancer caused some sufferers to 'become loathsome to themselves and to all about them'. Dale catalogued the various sedatives and narcotics and then turned to the 'new' medicines of ether and chloroform and their magical properties. Chloroform acts literally ' "as a charm", and cause[s] the wondering patient to give utterance to the most lively expressions of gratitude for the relief one has been able to afford him'.[198] Medical charisma was heightened by demonstrations of power over pain. Nowhere was this more clearly showcased than in the care of the dying.

Palliation of pain for the dying was pivotal, not just for patients, but for family and friends who had to witness their loved ones' suffering—it had been so since the eighteenth century. But by the 1880s, social fear of the pain of death had grown to such a degree that the physician William Munk published a treatise: *Euthanasia: or Medical Treatment in Aid of an Easy Death*. Munk's desire to make death as easy and painless as possible stemmed from his thoughtfulness and experience, commented the *Lancet*. Few doctors wrote on euthanasia; medical students were not taught the principles of managing death. Doctors must remember that much of their social position depended on 'their office as healers of the sick and ministers at the bedside', advised the *Lancet*.[199] Munk employed opiates freely, and promoted hypodermic injections of morphine: fears of addiction were irrelevant in such cases, he argued. (Legal restrictions on the sale of opiates had been introduced in 1868 in an attempt to tackle the problem of opiate addiction.) Stimulants like sherry, port, and brandy were useful, as was an appealing diet. Simple practical measures like limiting the number of visitors, choosing light bedclothes, and keeping the room fresh and light were of huge benefit.

But no amount of medical care, warned Munk (a Roman Catholic), could ease more than the physical suffering of disbelievers or agnostics: 'doubt and anxiety as to his future is all but sure to obtrude itself on his last conscious moments, disturb them, and render such an euthanasia as we contemplate, impossible.'[200] Munk's principles spread far and wide. Alice, sister of Henry and William James, was diagnosed with incurable breast cancer in 1891. 'Take all the morphia (or other forms of opium if that disagrees) you want, and don't be afraid of becoming an opium drunkard. What was opium created for except for such times as this,' advised William.[201] Withholding 'the inestimable boon afforded by opium in full doses' was a neglect of medical duty, ruled the *Lancet* in 1899.

Medical interest in terminal illness was not new. Devastated by his wife Elizabeth's death from cancer, William Marsden had set up the Cancer Hospital in Brompton, London, in 1851 for the poor. (It later became the Royal Marsden Hospital—the word cancer was thought to frighten and deter patients.) By the time the surgeon Herbert Snow (no relation to John) had joined its staff in 1876, Marsden had died, but his work was continuing. One of Marsden's interests had been to palliate cancer cases that were beyond surgical intervention. Snow took up the torch and promoted the use of opiates and cocaine. *The Palliative Treatment of Incurable Cancer* (1890) included an appendix on the use of the opium pipe. He was also famous for the Brompton cocktail—a mixture of morphine and cocaine—which relieved the pain of advanced cancer. As well as drugs, Snow stressed the benefits of good nursing and support from the hospital chaplaincy service. Nevertheless many patients continued to die in pain—some remained frightened to the end. Canadian physician William Osler studied 500 terminally ill patients finding that 'Ninety suffered great bodily pain or distress of one sort or another, 11 showed mental apprehension, 2 positive terror'. Osler, appointed as Professor of Medicine at Oxford in 1905, had caused a storm of controversy in his farewell speech to the Johns Hopkins University. Old age, he said, was worthless: 'Take the sum of human achievement in action, in science, in art, in literature—subtract the work of men above 40, and while we should miss great treasures, even priceless treasures, we would practically be where we are today.'[202] There was a solution. Osler reminded his audience of Anthony Trollope's futuristic novel, *The Fixed Period*, published in 1881 when Trollope was 66 years old. Trollope had looked forward to 1980 when, in an imaginary Australasian state, the narrator and main protagonist John Neverbend, president of the Empire of the South Pacific, masterminded a plan to avoid suffering, and save society the 'costliness' of old age: men above 67½ years of age were 'peacefully extinguished' by a dose of chloroform. Critics interpreted it as a dark joke: the reading public did not much care for the topic; only 877 copies were sold and the publisher, Blackwood, lost money. Osler interpreted the criticism to hail from his jokey reference to Trollope's idea of enforced euthanasia by chloroform, rather than his ageist views. But Trollope did not jest. A few months before his own death, he wrote to his brother Tom: 'the time has come upon me ... in which I should know that it were better that I were dead.'[203] Facing old age, Trollope perhaps, thought death a better option than earthly suffering.

New discoveries continued to cushion pain at all ages. Snow's innovative Brompton Cocktail was made possible by the discovery of cocaine, which was also used on its own as a local anaesthetic. Coca leaves were used in South America for their analgesic properties and the active ingredient—cocaine—was isolated in 1859. A young neurologist in Vienna—Sigmund Freud, who later became famous for his psychoanalytical work—experimented with cocaine on patients addicted to morphine in the 1880s. He also tried it himself for severe depression: 'a small dose lifted me to the heights in a wonderful fashion.' Cocaine was a 'magical substance' which deserved a song of praise, he waxed lyrically.[204] In 1884 Freud asked his friend Carl Koller, an eye surgeon, to do some experiments with cocaine. Koller had already begun to search for a local anaesthetic because of the risks of ether and chloroform in eye surgery. Operations often required the patient to hold the eye still, which unconscious patients could not do, and post-anaesthetic vomiting could put undue pressure on the eyeball and prejudice the effectiveness of the surgery. Koller gave a solution of cocaine to a friend who remarked on the instant numbness of his tongue. It was not the first time this effect had been noted, but for Koller it was a eureka moment. He applied cocaine to frogs and found that after only a minute, the frog allowed its cornea to be touched and manipulated without any reflex action. Rabbits and dogs responded similarly. He used it himself and found that the anaesthesia could last for around half an hour. Cocaine was rapidly taken up in eye surgery and methods were devised for injecting it subcutaneously for other minor operations. As well as a local anaesthetic, cocaine proved beneficial for patients with cancerous growths: the usual treatment was to burn the growths off using caustic agents; an initial application of cocaine to the site diminished the pain. Meanwhile, research into salicylic acids (originally derived from willow bark and long known for their analgesic effects) attempted to eliminate the dangerous side effects of irritation to the stomach lining. The chemist Felix Hoffmann, working for German pharmaceutical company Bayer, produced acetylsalicylic acid in 1897. Marketed as aspirin from 1899, it became the most used and best known analgesic of all time.

Old understandings of pain as purposeful still bobbed on the medical horizon but were scornfully rebuffed. 'Pain never comes where it can serve no good purpose. Pain is eminently merciful,' declaimed H. Cameron Gillies in a series of articles, *The Life-Saving Value of Pain and Disease*, published in 1887. Doctors across the country took up their pens in protest: 'what daring presumption it must be to attempt to abolish that much-disguised blessing by the use of anaesthetics'; 'pain is distinctly harmful … it may turn the scales in the favour of death'; 'pain is a universal human legacy. It is the penalty we pay for our high state of development. It is what generations of medical men in all climes have striven with all their strength and knowledge to lessen or to annul'; Gillies's views were 'so strangely at variance with universal experience, no less than with common sense'. Arguments about the value of pain were out of kilter with 1880s thinking, particularly in regard to terminal illness. 'Is this the grim comfort [Gillies] would bring to a suffering women tortured slowly to death by a sloughing scirrhus of the breast, or to a man, made almost inhuman and killed by inches by the slow yet sure ravages of a rodent ulcer?', expostulated W. J. Collins.[205] Pain which had seemed intrinsic to the human condition in the 1840s—'pain is … instrumental to good', Harriet Martineau had decided in 1844—was now an alien force which undermined man's very humanity.[206]

That palliation of pain was integral to the foundations of a civilized society was at the root of many of the social changes which occurred during Queen Victoria's reign. In the eighteenth century the new humanitarianism had ignited reform of cruelty to animals; in the nineteenth century it focused on the gritty issue of vivisection—the use of animals for experiments. The first piece of legislation to protect animals against cruelty was instigated in 1822 by 'Humanity Dick', nickname of Irish MP Richard Martin, and supported by a small group of reformers including William Wilberforce. Known as Martin's Act, the Cruel Treatment of Cattle Act introduced penalties for cruelty to cattle and horses in markets, slaughterhouses, towns, and countryside. Two years later, the same groups of reformers established the Society for the Prevention of Cruelty to Animals. It gained Royal status in 1840 and by 1841 employed five inspectors who travelled around Britain bringing offenders to justice. In 1835, the Cruelty to Animals Act had banned cock-fighting, bear-baiting with dogs, and badger-baiting. But old habits died hard. Bull-baiting was the 'most barbarous act I ever saw. It was [a] young bull and had very little notion of tossing the dogs, which tore his ears and the skin off his face in shreds,' noted Shropshire man James Gryce in 1878.

The RSPCA's work in prosecuting offenders was widely supported. An RSPCA officer was called in by Charles Darwin in 1853 to take action against a man in his village for cruelty to carthorses. When he was a student in pre-anaesthetic days Darwin's intense sensitivity to pain had caused him to flee from the operating theatre. It also caused problems in his research. To iron out details of breeding and inheritance in his evolution theory, later published as the *Origin of Species* (1859), Darwin developed a passion for pigeons, watching them live and breed, then skeletonizing them to 'watch their insides'. But how to kill a pigeon? Darwin tried chloroform but it took too long, and he could not bear to watch their slow death. In the end, potassium cyanide in a bottle, which gave off prussic acid gas, was the quickest way. But however humanely death was achieved, it remained the 'black deed' of murder. Nor could Darwin cope with soaking the corpses to rot the flesh before boiling the carcases: it 'made my servant and myself ... retch so violently, that we were compelled to desist'.[207] Pragmatically he despatched the dead birds to be skeletonized professionally.

Distaste for vivisection had long been part of British culture. Anatomist Charles Bell, whose 1820s work on the brain identified specific sites for specific sensory and motor functions, performed as few vivisection experiments as possible, preferring to progress his work through observation. In Britain, most physiological research was carried out in the homes of researchers like John Snow, rather than in universities. Physiologists remained low profile until concern about their activities escalated in the early 1860s in a series of intense and hostile medical and public debates. For some, anaesthesia solved the moral dilemmas of vivisection. Benjamin Ward Richardson, friend and biographer of John Snow, researched the physiology of anaesthesia by experimenting on animals but gave them chloroform. No charge of cruelty could be sustained if anaesthesia saved the animals pain, he argued. But anxieties continued to torment experimentalists like Darwin: 'You ask about my opinion on vivisection. I quite agree that it is justifiable for real investigations on physiology; but not for mere damnable and detestable curiosity. It is a subject which makes me sick with horror, so I will not say another word about it, else I shall not sleep to-night,' he wrote to Professor Ray Lankester in 1871.[208]

Matters boiled up in 1874 at a meeting of the British Medical Association when the French neurologist Valentin Magnan's demonstration of the effects of absinthe on two sensible dogs provoked a prosecution. In 1875 a Royal Commission was set up to investigate the matter, and the Society for the Protection of Animals Liable to Vivisection was established by Frances Power Cobbe, social reformer and leading figure in the British women's suffrage campaign. As the guardian angels of social morality, women, of course, were ideally placed to lead the debate. In a letter to her brother, Dante Gabriel Rossetti, in 1875 the poet Christina Rossetti wrote that she believed anaesthesia had resolved the issue of vivisection:

> I used to believe with you that chloroform was so largely used as to do away with the horror of Vivisection: but a friend has so urged the subject upon me, & has sent me so many printed documents alleg-

ing & apparently establishing the contrary, that I have felt impelled
to do what little I could to gain help against what … is cruelty of a
revolting magnitude.[209]

Some resolution was achieved by the 1876 Cruelty to Animals Act,
which legalized vivisection under certain conditions: licensed doctors, licensed premises, the use of anaesthesia with special excep-
tions, and annual reports. The flames died down, but the embers
continued to glow. Correspondence in *The Times* between Darwin
and Cobbe in 1881 revealed a continuing impasse. Darwin had responded to a request from Swedish Professor Holmgren from Upsala
and stated his opinion that English physiologists had been falsely
accused of cruelty in 1875 though he feared that 'in some parts of
Europe little regard is paid to the sufferings of animals'.[210] Cobbe
challenged the accuracy of his view and iterated the moral dangers
for all nationalities: 'What shall it profit a man if he gain the whole
world of knowledge and lose his own heart and conscience?'[211]

Cobbe's protest that inflicting pain on defenceless creatures jeop-
ardized the moral basis of a civilized society had been part of the earlier arguments against animal cruelty—as indeed it was in reforms
of slavery and prisons. Butchers who slaughtered and prepared meat
were 'callous to the feeling of the animal creation': daily witness of
painful animal deaths made them 'deficient in sympathy for their
fellow-creatures', wrote one physician to the Lancet in 1840.[212] But
morality could be safeguarded by making death painless. Slaughter
animals by tying bags of Indian-rubber cloth over mouths and nostrils and administer carbon dioxide gas, suggested the correspondent. Forty years later, Benjamin Ward Richardson pioneered new
methods of painless extinction at the Home for Lost Dogs where a
chamber was charged with a mixture of carbon dioxide and chloroform. Whilst in a profound sleep, the dogs passed from life to death
without experiencing pain or consciousness of their state.

Figure 13 This 1872 Punch cartoon satirizes the assumed incompetency of female doctors against the surgical prowess of males and also suggests the surgeon's superiority over the anaesthetist. The caption reads: 'Doctor Evangeline: "By the bye, Mr Sawyer, are you engaged tomorrow afternoon? I have a rather ticklish operation to perform— an amputation, you know." Mr Sawyer: "I shall be very happy to do it for you." Doctor Evangeline: "O, no, not *that!* But will you kindly come and administer the chloroform for me?"'

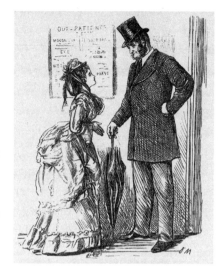

Painless surgery dissipated moral concerns about the role of the surgeon and his infliction of pain on patients. It also swept away one of the strongest arguments against women entering medicine and being associated with the pain and brutality of surgery, although the idea of a female surgeon remained novel for many years. Many Victorians continued to view surgery as a distasteful spectacle for the female sex—even vaccinations. 'What will not women do nowadays! Mrs Heimann with her friend ... actually went to the Pasteur Institute and *saw the operation performed* on over 70 patients,' exclaimed Christina Rossetti in 1889.[213]

Concern for morality was at the heart of the reforms of the penal system which sought to eliminate violence from the public arena, and so we return to where we began. In the years before Michael Barrett's hanging, repugnance of the spectacle of public executions grew. Novelist William Thackeray's 1840 responses to the 'hideous debauchery' of a public execution which left him with 'an extraordinary feeling of terror and shame' that he had been 'abetting an act of frightful wickedness and violence, performed by a set of men against one of their fellows', were reiterated almost a decade later by Charles Dickens.[214] For Dickens, the most abhorrent aspect of the execution he witnessed at Horsemonger Gaol in November 1849 was 'the wickedness and levity of the immense crowd'. As dawn broke, sunlight

> gilded thousands upon thousands of upturned faces, so inexpress-
> ibly odious in their brutal mirth or callousness, that a man had cause
> to feel ashamed of the shape he wore, and to shrink from himself,
> as fashioned in the image of the Devil. When the two miserable
> creatures who attracted all this ghastly sight about them were turned
> quivering into the air, there was no more emotion, no more pity, no
> more thought that two immortal souls had gone to judgement, no
> more restraint in any of the previous obscenities, than if the name of
> Christ had never been heard in this world, and there were no beliefs
> among men but that they perished like the beasts.[215]

For Thackeray and Dickens the root of the problem was not so much the act of violence per se, but its corrupting influence on those who watched the executions. In other words, witnessing the inflic- tion of physical suffering was dangerous because it encouraged the transgression of moral boundaries. Removing executions from the public arena became a social compromise. Public scenes of brutality and violence were cleared from towns and cities, but capital punish- ment remained the ultimate social deterrent against crime—behind prison walls, the brutal taking of life continued.

In Maidstone prison, on 14 August 1868, 18-year-old Thomas Wells was executed for shooting the local stationmaster. Unlike Barrett's hanging, Wells's ordeal took place out of public view. It prompted *The Times*, which had previously opposed the abolition campaign, to comment that such reforms were 'hard to realise before they are made, but which, once made, seem so simple and unobjectionable that they are treated almost as a matter of course'.[216] However, its commentary on punishment in December 1894 suggested soul-searching continued: 'We are not all so sure as we once were of the good effects of a residence in prison, or of the genesis of crime. We do not hang or imprison a man with the self-complacency and sense of self-righteousness of our fathers.'[217] Public distaste for witnessing any form of physical punishment grew to such an extent that there were protests over handcuffed prisoners being marched through streets, or taken on the railways: 'The spectacle of handcuffed women in a public place is certainly unusual, and revolting to the feelings of most people,' said the *Western Mail* in 1899.[218] The new generation of Victorians who knew anaesthesia to be a routine blessing of modern society could no longer stomach physical suffering in any form. It was a 'strange moral transformation', remarked the psychologist and philosopher William James, brother of Henry, the novelist. By 1902 'we no longer think that we are called upon to face physical pain with equanimity. It is not expected of a man that he should either endure it or inflict much of it, and to listen to the recitals of cases of it makes our flesh creep morally as well as physically,' noted James.[219] Distaste of physical suffering had been at the heart of an upheaval in the Church of England which uprooted old ideas and meanings of pain in religious doctrine.

The schism had first appeared in the 1840s when Charles Darwin and George Eliot among others began to doubt the use of deliberately inflicted pain in religious doctrine. The 'crisis of faith', as it was called at the time, is often explained as a natural consequence of evolutionary philosophies which suggested that deterministic mechanisms like 'natural selection' and the 'survival of the fittest' shaped the world. But doubters were more occupied with the role of physical punishment. Images of Hell as a place where the physical torture of burning flames lasted an eternity seemed at odds with the promise of a loving and beneficient God. How could such dreadful suffering be Divinely sanctioned? Darwin struggled for some years with Christian notions of everlasting punishment and original sin. The death of his young daughter, Annie, in April 1851 was the final straw. She was 'in simple truth angelic' and died 'as tranquilly as a little angel', he said.[220] From that point Darwin acknowledged his loss of belief although it remained a permanent sorrow, dividing him from his wife, Emma, who kept faith with Christian beliefs.

By the 1860s public antipathy to physical suffering was intense. Charles Voysey, Church of England curate who was charged with heresy, and later founded the Theistic Church in London, exclaimed:

> I am literally besieged with letters pressing me for an answer to the questions, Why should there be so much apparently needless suffering in the world? How can we, in the presence of these painful facts, believe in the existence and sovereign control of a good God? On every hand such and kindred discussions are raised. One hardly ever touches the subject of Religion without the conversation drifting rapidly to this central and vital enquiry.[221]

Voysey's case was only one of several: F. D. Maurice was tried for refusing to teach the doctrine of eternal damnation—strongly associated with physical pain and punishment—to his students at King's College, London.

The deep transformation in religious understandings of pain was addressed by Herbert Spencer in his autobiography, published in 1904. The common view of God in the 1840s, explained Spencer, was 'a deity who is pleased with the singing of his praises, and angry with the beings he has made when they fail to tell him perpetually of his greatness'. At that time, he continued, 'it had not become manifest to me how absolutely and immeasurably unjust it would be that for Adam's disobedience (which might have caused a harsh man to discharge his servant), all Adam's descendants should be damned ... [God was] a being who calmly looks on while myriads of his creatures are suffering eternal torments.'²²² In Spencer's lifetime, pain had been recast in Christian doctrine as a form of spiritual, rather than physical suffering. Hell had become a place of moral torment rather than bodily anguish. The anaesthetic process itself emerged as a means of spiritual enlightenment. American naturalist, poet, and author Henry D. Thoreau had breathed ether at his dentist's in 1851 and found it to be revelatory. 'You are told that it will make you unconscious,' he wrote in his journal,

> but no one can imagine what it is to be unconscious—how far removed from the state of consciousness & all that we call 'this world' until he has experienced it. The value of the experiment is that it does give you experience of an interval as between one life and another ... You expand like a seed in the ground. You exist in your roots—like a tree in the winter. If you have an inclination to travel take the ether—you go beyond the furthest star.²²³

During the 1860s 'the anaesthetic revelation' became established as a philosophical phenomenon, largely thanks to American philosopher and poet Benjamin Paul Blood. After breathing nitrous oxide for dentistry in 1860, Blood devoted his life to analysing the mystical fallout of his experience and published *The Anaesthetic Revelation and the Gist of Philosophy* (1874). Patients who experienced the phenomenon regained consciousness with an awareness that they had 'known the oldest truth'. No longer would 'human theories as to the origin, meaning, or destiny of the race' have meaning: anaesthesia had put these individuals beyond instruction in 'spiritual things', explained Blood.²²⁴ English poet and literary critic John Addington

Symonds agreed: 'at the moment of recovery from anaesthesia, just then, *before Starting on life*, I catch, so to speak, ... a glimpse of the eternal process just in the act of starting.'[225] Fiction too explored the capacity of anaesthesia to generate mysticism. The narrator in Guy de Maupassant's story *Afloat*, published in 1888, breathed ether to relieve migraine:

> I noticed that my head was no longer hurting ... I was not asleep, I was awake; I was understanding, I was feeling, I was reasoning with an accuracy, a depth, a power which were extraordinary ... It seemed to me that I had tasted of the Tree of Knowledge, that all the mysteries had been unveiled, so much did I find myself under the sway of a new, strange, irrefutable logic.[226]

Philosopher William James analysed the interplay between anaesthesia and spirituality. Anaesthesia kaleidoscoped all layers of consciousness into one whole, resolving conflicts and contradictions, and providing deep and lasting insights into the meaning of life: 'depth beyond depth of truth seems revealed to the inhaler,' he noted in *The Varieties of Religious Experience* (1902). A century earlier, Davy and his associates' claims for the enlightening powers of nitrous oxide had been sidelined as dangerously radical. Through the nineteenth century, breathing chemicals had metamorphosed, not just into a routine method of surgical pain relief, but into a pathway to transcendental knowledge and the oldest truths of the universe.

The reign of Queen Victoria thus drew to a close with anaesthesia, emblem of humanitarianism, embedded in surgery, and the revolutionary philosophies which drove its establishment legitimized in the structures and practices of society. For Victorians, saving pain had become a medical and social goal, consonant with the very essence of modern civilization.

8

· · · ·

INTO THE TWENTIETH
CENTURY AND BEYOND

Victorians poised on the brink of a new century considered anaesthesia as one of the best fruits of their times. In chloroform's
jubilee year, the Duke of Cambridge opened a new operating theatre at St George's Hospital: nothing during the reign of Queen Victoria had made as much progress as medical and surgical science, he
said. Four years later, the Victorian era ended with the death of the
Queen in 1901, and a new reign began. About-to-be Edwardians,
reading of the postponement of Edward's coronation on account of
his suffering an abscess in the appendix, did not, perhaps, appreciate
that had Victoria, rather than Edward suffered the same condition,
matters may have been very different. Appendicitis was not within
the medical lexicon in 1837. Presenting with the same symptoms
as her son, the diagnosis of the future Queen's malady would have
been gastric seizure, or cramp of the bowel. In such cases, an operation was too risky. It was a case of watching and waiting. With luck,
the abscess might have resolved after several weeks' illness. If not,
sepsis could have set in—the end might have been fatal and could
have changed the course of history.

Edward had the advantages of anaesthesia, antisepsis, and new
surgical knowledge. Joseph Lister's introduction of antisepsis tech-

niques in the 1860s had allowed the surgical repertoire to blossom and the chest, abdomen, and brain became new surgical sites. Operations like herniotomies, removal of cancer of the rectum or stomach, and appendicitis were new surgical solutions to old medical problems: 'there has scarcely been anything more remarkable in the way of medicine at the close of the nineteenth century than the sudden appearance of the disease now known as appendicitis,' stated Frederick Treves, surgeon and Professor of Surgery at the London hospital, in the Cavendish Lecture, delivered on 20 June 1902.[227] Four days later Treves drained Edward's appendix abscess whilst Frederick Hewitt, anaesthetist at the London and St George's hospitals, administered a mixture of chloroform and ether. Publicized widely, the operation drew little response apart from messages from well-wishers. Edward's recovery was swift: he was crowned King on 9 August 1902.

Victorians had just cause for pride: anaesthesia was given to any patient—royal or pleb—and painful operations were becoming part of Western history. But new operations like appendectomy demanded new anaesthetic conditions: it was almost impossible for a surgeon to close an abdominal wound if muscle reflexes had not been suspended and the guts writhed with a life of their own under his hands. To suspend muscle reflex required deep anaesthesia but large doses of agents like chloroform or ether were considered risky in the elderly, and in some cases of chronic disease. John Snow's practice of specialist anaesthesia had been taken up following his death in 1858 by a small group of followers, most notably Joseph Clover. Present at Liston's first use of ether at University College Hospital in 1846, Clover later developed a wide range of anaesthetic apparatus and shared Snow's skills in reassuring nervous patients. From the 1870s onwards, in London hospitals and the larger provincial institutions, specialist anaesthetists combined anaesthetic agents—

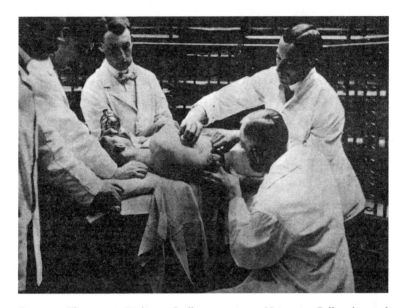

Figure 14 The surgeon Rickman Godlee operating at University College hospital in 1899 whilst a Clover inhaler or modification is used to administer the anaesthetic. Godlee had been highly criticized in 1884 for removing a brain tumour from a young man who subsequently died from complications.

nitrous oxide, ether, and chloroform—in various sequences to surmount the problems created by the new surgery. But in most parts of Britain, non-specialists continued to administer chloroform on a cloth. Our story concludes by moving into the twentieth century and beyond to consider how these many challenges were resolved against the backdrop of two world wars and, in Britain, the establishment of the National Health Service.

Treves and his peers acknowledged fully the debt surgery owed to anaesthesia: it had 'greatly extended the domain of surgery by rendering possible operations which before could only have been dreamt about, and by allowing elaborate measures to be carried out step by step', explained Treves.[228] Some commentators took a different view. The 'craze' for surgery had created needless operations, protested George Bernard Shaw in *Doctor's Dilemma* (1906). Patients had been duped, by their own fallibility, as well as by surgeons, to believe that 'chloroform has made surgery painless'. Chloroform had become a new tool in the medical armoury, allowing surgeons to extract money from patients. Sir Patrick, Shaw's protagonist, told of the Walpole medical dynasty:

> The father used to snip off the ends of people's uvulas for fifty guineas, and paint throats with caustic every day for a year at two guineas a time. His brother-in-law extirpated tonsils for two hundred guineas until he took up women's cases at double the fees. Cutler himself worked hard at anatomy to find something fresh to operate on; and at last he got hold of something he calls the nuciform sac, which he's made quite the fashion. People pay him five hundred guineas to cut it out. They might as well get their hair cut for all the difference it makes; but I suppose they feel important after it. You can't go out to dinner now without your neighbour bragging to you of some useless operation or other.

Shaw's cynicism may have been particularly hard-edged but it ignored the persistent worry of anaesthesia: unexplained chloroform death.

Chloroform, the riskiest of the three anaesthetics discovered during the nineteenth century, remained the most popular. Nitrous oxide, introduced as an anaesthetic in 1868, was the mainstay of dentistry; its quickly produced, short-acting effects suited brief extractions. Ether, reintroduced into Britain during the 1870s, remained the province of the specialist. The unwavering popularity of chloroform is one of the most interesting questions in the history of anaesthesia. Chloroform was the easiest anaesthetic to give and the 'rag and bottle' method—chloroform dropped on to a simple face mask—suited most situations. This was a key consideration as most anaesthetics were given by general practitioners without specialist training. Medical and public concern about chloroform fatalities was strong. Doctors were acute to the professional ordeal of having a patient die under chloroform. Deaths under anaesthetics were subject to coroners' inquests and the doctor who gave the anaesthetic had to take the stand and defend his actions: 'if the patient dies from the anaesthetic, the man who has administered the poison has killed him, and, therefore, in a sense, it is for him to justify what he has done,' noted Manchester coroner E. A. Gibson.[229] These cases were regularly publicized in newspapers. Nevertheless, in nineteenth-century Britain no doctor was charged with anaesthetic malpractice after a chloroform fatality. The great British stoicism inured patients to the risks of anaesthesia: fear of pain outstripped worries of dying under chloroform and fatalities were tolerated as a worrying, though inherent risk of anaesthesia. Across the Atlantic patients differed, particularly in the Northern states. Boston surgeons had no illusions about patients' litigious predilections: medical malpractice suits against surgeons were common and using a riskier anaesthetic—chloroform—when ether was known to be safer could not be defended. The Southern states were more British in their attitudes to risk and chloroform continued to be used. But worldwide, understandings of chloroform death remained unresolved and old Scottish–London rivalries as to whether chloroform poisoned the heart or damaged the respiration configured the debate. Matters came to a head in the Indian state of Hyderabad, more famous generally for its entrancing landscape enhanced with mosques and minarets, bazaars and bridges.

In 1884 the British army surgeon Edward Lawrie had been appointed principal to Hyderabad's medical school (now known as Osmania Medical College) and four years later set up a commission to investigate chloroform death. Lawrie, disciple of the Scottish view that respiration not the heart was the focus of chloroform death, chose a prize-giving, attended by the Duke and Duchess of Connaught, to attack London views that chloroform killed by its action on the heart. Results of the commission's 128 experiments on dogs suggested that respiration was the vulnerable function under chloroform. Chloroform deaths will continue, stressed Lawrie, until the London medical community changes its principles—or swaps to ether. Lawrie's challenge was picked up by the *Lancet*, who chose Dr Thomas Lauder Brunton, Edinburgh graduate and physician at St Bartholomew's, to visit Hyderabad and review Lawrie's claims. Brunton's conclusions may have been foregone given his already published view that chloroform killed through direct action on the heart. The first telegram suggested otherwise: 'Four hundred and ninety dogs, horses, monkeys, goats, cats and rabbits used. ... All records photographed. ... Results most instructive. Danger from chloroform is asphyxia or overdose; none whatever heart direct.'[230] London remained stubborn. 'We thought that it would be well to supplement the work of that Commission as far as possible by a consideration of the results arrived at by clinical observation,' said the *Lancet*. It asked Dudley Wilmot Buxton, one of London's specialist anaesthetists, to supervise a survey of practice. All British hospitals with ten or more beds, and larger hospitals across Europe, the Colonies, the USA, and India were sent a questionnaire: 'What anaesthetic do you usually employ, and how? Can you give particulars of any deaths? Agents used? Apparatus? Did heart or respiration stop first?' were some of the questions. Replies were gathered within a year; analysis of results took two more. There were few surprises. In Britain, chloroform topped the charts, usually given with a handkerchief or cloth: it was also the most popular anaesthetic in private practice. Chloroform mortality remained higher than that of ether. In India and the Tropics, chloroform was the main anaesthetic but inexplicably appeared to have a mortality rate lower than that in Britain. Few changed their practice.

In 1901, the British Medical Association established a chloroform committee under the leadership of Augustus Waller, lecturer on physiology at St Mary's Hospital medical school. This stimulated the Oxford chemist Vernon Harcourt to devise an apparatus which limited the dosage of chloroform to safe levels. Yet deaths still continued. In 1911, the physiologist A. Goodman Levy's experiments on cats under chloroform provided the missing link in the chloroform death puzzle by showing that ventricular fibrillation could occur during light anaesthesia: 'this form of syncope is extremely sudden in onset, and the patient is plunged from life into death in an instant ... The heart-beat then ceases absolutely suddenly, the face is blanched white, the pupils dilate extremely, and drops of sweat may form on the face and body,' wrote Levy.[231] The only way to avert disaster was to pay constant attention to the pulse; an irregular or flickering pulse was the only sign of approaching danger.

Levy's work was significant, not just for anaesthesia but for the rapidly developing specialty of cardiology. It did not change practice though. Some anaesthetists familiarized themselves with Levy's findings—he addressed the 1912 annual BMA meeting and the Royal Society of Medicine in 1914—but for most, Levy's animal experiments bore little relation to clinical practice and chloroform's intricacies remained enigmatic. In 1922 Levy summarized his findings in *Chloroform Anaesthesia*: a work which would hopefully enlighten 'the whole subject of the effects of anaesthetics', wrote *The Times* medical correspondent.[232] Most anaesthetic teachers taught students to avoid chloroform for the induction of anaesthesia, countered St George's Hospital anaesthetist, Joseph Blomfield. Fatalities continued to make headlines. In 1923, one London hospital reported forty-two chloroform deaths in a matter of eight weeks, and the Poplar

Hospital, founded by Samuel Gurney, banker and philanthropist, to care for those injured on the docks, suffered three fatalities on one day. 'Week after week the chloroform holocaust goes on,' despaired one correspondent to the *British Medical Journal*.[233] The American Medical Association's Committee of Anaesthesia had concluded in 1912 that chloroform was too risky to be justified.

Instruction in anaesthesia had been included on the General Medical Council's list of required subjects since 1911. But few doctors built upon this basic training and the specialist anaesthetist remained a rare creature. In London, the Society of Anaesthetists attracted forty members when it was created in 1893. Before the First World War there were fewer than ten anaesthetic specialists in the USA. There, most anaesthetics were given by nurses. The dearth of anaesthetic skills became clear during the First World War and prompted Arthur Guedel to introduce a simple way of teaching safe anaesthesia. Guedel had graduated from the University of Indiana in 1908, set up in general practice, and developed a growing interest in anaesthesia. At the outbreak of the Great War, Guedel joined the American Expeditionary Force in the spa town of Vittel in France's Vosges Mountains, and found a 'deplorable lack of knowledge of anaesthesia'. Base hospitals of the war zones were staffed by nurses and enlisted men from the army medical corps with little or no medical training. Guedel's solution was simple but effective. He created a chart which showed how the body responded to ether at different degrees of anaesthesia. In one sense it was a visual representation of Snow's earlier teachings on the anaesthetic process. The administrator could check the patient's respiration, eyeball activity, pupils, eyelid reflex, and so on against the chart and feel confident that the anaesthetic was proceeding safely. Guedel's short frequent visits to base hospitals meant he could troubleshoot problems and train new personnel. He became notorious: he 'blows in here every day or two, like a wild Indian, on a motorcycle', said one medical officer at the unit in Vittel.[234] Most anaesthetists returned home at the end of the war certain that something should be done about anaesthesia, noted University of North Carolina Professor of Surgery, David A. Davis. The war also stimulated the development of new anaesthetic techniques.

Trench warfare produced horrific injuries to the face and neck and many of the wounded soldiers were evacuated from the Somme to England. New Zealander Harold Gillies, trained in medicine at Cambridge and St Bartholomews' Hospital, served with the Royal Army Medical Corps and persuaded officers at the Cambridge Military Hospital, Aldershot, of the need for specialist reconstructive surgery for soldiers with facial injuries. Over time numbers of patients outran the space and a new hospital was built in Sidcup, Kent, sponsored by Queen Mary. It was the first in Britain to specialize in facial injuries and Gillies's repertoire expanded rapidly to include burns, limb injuries, and congenital malformations. Over 5,000 wounded soldiers were treated between 1917 and 1925. Anaesthesia posed a particular challenge: patients often had to remain upright during operations as injuries to the face and neck created respiratory difficulties and in some cases it was almost impossible to administer anaesthetic using a mask or inhaler. Ivan Magill and Stanley Rowbotham, medical officers during the war, were posted to the hospital in 1919. They were, remembered Rowbotham, 'precipitously and without training plunged into the task of administering some of the most difficult and hazardous anaesthetics that one could meet'.[235] Ether, administered through the rectum, was one solution to the problem of having little access to the face but it was very difficult to control the depth of anaesthesia: some patients took as long as twenty-four hours to come round after an operation, said Rowbotham. This set of problems stimulated Magill and

Rowbotham to develop endotracheal intubation. Administering anaesthesia through a tube fed down the patient's trachea avoided the need for mouthpieces or facemasks. Collaboration between the anaesthetists and the manufacturers ensured that a range of tubes in graduated sizes was produced to fit all shapes and sizes of patients. Ingenious technology solved the anaesthetic problems but the legacy of disfigurement remained. War casualties were issued with blue uniforms for wear during their hospital stays. This outfit was a British 'badge of honour, which ensures respect everywhere' affirmed the Black Cat cigarette card which featured a blue-uniformed 'Tommy' in 1919. But those suffering facial injuries were more likely to encounter repulsion, fear, and pity. Some of the Sidcup wounded shrouded their injuries with thin metal facemasks; benches on the route between Sidcup and the hospital were painted blue to warn local people that they might encounter some of the disfigured soldiers on the benches. The injuries were also immortalized in art by Henry Tonks, who trained as a surgeon then abandoned medicine in favour of art, becoming Professor of Fine Art at the University of London in 1917.

In the aftermath of the First World War new discoveries began to ameliorate some of the knotty problems of anaesthesia, particularly muscle relaxation. The solution came from curare, used for centuries as arrow poisons in South America and well known to doctors. But it did not come rapidly.

In the 1800s, early experimenters like the surgeon Benjamin Brodie found curare paralysed animals but so long as respiration was maintained it did not kill them. French physiologist Claude Bernard's experiments in the 1860s showed how curare's action was specific and local: it caused muscle paralysis by inhibiting the nerve impulse. It was found to be useful in the treatment of hydrophobia, tetanus, and strychnine poisoning. Arthur Lawen in Leipzig used small doses of curare on anaesthetized patients in 1912; New Zealand anaesthetist Francis Percival de Caux, trained at St Bartholomew's in the 1920s, found curare a useful conjunct to nitrous oxide anaesthesia, but neither published the experiments widely. The production of a standardized form of curare by New York pharmaceutical company E. R. Squibb was inspired by Richard C. Gill's quest to relieve the symptoms of multiple sclerosis. Gill had lived for several years on the eastern slopes of the Andes in Ecuador and was skilled in the intricacies of Indian herbal medicine, winning the confidence of local witch-doctors and watching them make poisoned arrows. Diagnosed with multiple sclerosis in the 1930s, Gill suffered spastic paralysis and discussed the potential of curare with Walter Freeman, his neurologist. Gill's burning desire to return to the jungle to collect supplies of curare drove an intensive period of rehabilitation and he set out on his expedition in May 1938. He returned five months later with around seventy-five plant specimens and 12 kg of curare. Eventually Squibb agreed to purchase the curare and standardize it: it appeared on the market in 1941 under the name Intocostrin.

Physician Lewis Wright, trainee of Ernest Rovenstine, Professor of Anaesthesia in New York, spotted Intocostrin's potential while working at Squibb. But early results were disappointing. Stuart Cullen, anaesthetist in Iowa City, trialled it on dogs but found it caused severe respiratory depression and the onset of asphyxia; in New York, E. M. Papper, later Chairman of the Anaesthesia department, used cats but they died, apparently from asthma. Surprisingly, given the litigious nature of the American public, Rovenstine agreed that Papper should try Intocostrin on patients. But the patients suffered such respiratory paralysis that they had to be manually ventilated overnight. Intocostrin was also being used to alleviate the severe muscle spasms caused by electroconvulsive therapy and the work of the psychiatrist A. E. Bennett in Nebraska encouraged Harold

Griffith, head of anaesthesia at the Homeopathic Hospital in Montreal, to pursue its possibilities. 'I argued to myself that if it did not kill Dr Bennett's patients it could hardly do any harm to ours, because the major danger would be respiratory paralysis and even at that time anaesthetists were accustomed to maintaining controlled respiration over long periods, so I asked Dr Wright to send me some Intocostrin,' Griffith later explained.[236] He and his assistant Enid Johnson found Intocostrin to be successful on patients under light cyclopropane anaesthesia. Word spread.

Ralph Waters, first professor of anaesthesia in the USA, trialled Intocostrin with nitrous oxide anaesthesia and again found it worked well. In Britain, anaesthetist Helen Barnes, who worked with the Emergency Medical Service in London, learnt about Intocostrin's application in psychiatry. She had the idea of using it to relax the laryngeal muscles and ease the process of intubation. Obtaining a sample from Squibb, Barnes experimented, not on a patient, but on herself. Two colleagues injected Intocostrin: 'My sensations were dramatic,' she wrote to the *Lancet*. 'At once my vision became blurred and almost "blacked out".' Drooping eyelids caused by the paralysis 'became very oppressive, and was accompanied by extreme prostration, fatigue, a sense of impending death, and a transient sensation of constriction in the throat'.[237] Nevertheless, her pulse and blood pressure remained steady though respiration became shallow. She recovered without any ill effects and tried intubating patients lightly anaesthetized with nitrous oxide, ether, and thiopental after injecting Intocostrin and spraying cocaine on the larynx. 'Is not modern anaesthesia getting out of hand?', was one response to her letter. The writer feared that Intocostrin might tempt less experienced anaesthetists to rely on drugs rather than skills to underpin their work. Intubation was 'a manoeuvre that only extreme gentleness and patience, coupled with a thorough knowledge of the anatomy and physiology of the larynx, can encompass successfully'.[238] As it turned out, the problems created by muscle relaxants lay elsewhere.

By 1945 Squibb was manufacturing around 100,000 doses of Intocostrin a month, most of which was used throughout the USA: UK anaesthestists turned to D-tubocurarine, an alkaloid developed by Wellcome and Co. which seemed to give equally good results although it required a far lower dose. But some anaesthetists believed muscle relaxants produced unconsciousness as well as paralysis. Utah University's Professor of Pharmacology, Louis S. Goodman, proved otherwise by testing Intocostrin on himself and reporting his experience in 1947. At the same time in the UK, Frederick Prescott, clinical research director at the Wellcome Research Institution, and anaesthetists Geoffrey Organe and Stanley Rowbotham analysed the effects of D-tubocurarine. Prescott was the guinea pig. It was terrifying: 'to be conscious yet paralysed and unable to breathe is a very unpleasant experience,' he said.[239] Strips of adhesive plaster torn from a hairy part of Prescott's body produced considerable pain and proved that muscle relaxants did not provide pain relief. Although the notion that muscle relaxants acted as analgesics was quickly quashed, some patients suffered unbearably because of an interruption with the anaesthetic supply; one patient reported in 1950:

> I remember going to sleep after your injection into my arm, but some time later was wakened by the most excruciating pain in my tummy. It felt as if my whole insides were being pulled out; I wanted to cry but I couldn't move any part of me, I heard the doctors talking about the gallbladder, then I went to sleep again.[240]

Muscle relaxants were a crucial breakthrough, vastly improving operating conditions for surgeons. Keith Sykes and John Bunker observe that those anaesthetists 'who mastered the new knowledge found that they were in complete control of the patient and capable of coping with the expanding horizons of the surgical specialties'.[241] Patients' experience of anaesthesia was revolutionized by new short-acting barbiturates. Given intravenously, these produced sleep within seconds and the unpleasantness of inhaling pungent anaesthetics was lost in unconsciousness. One of the most effective drugs was Evipan (hexibarbitone) introduced in 1934 in Germany by Dusseldorf clinical pharmacologist Helmutt Weese. Pentothal (thiopentone, now known as thiopental) was introduced in the USA in 1935. Few patients though benefited from these new drugs until after the Second World War. Why? Numbers of anaesthetists remained low in Britain during the interwar period though the number of GPs augmenting their practice with anaesthetic work at cottage hospitals or nursing homes increased. The gulf remained between the specially trained anaesthetist who manipulated a range of anaesthetics and techniques, tailored to individual patient and surgical requirements, and the majority of administrators who continued to rely on chloroform and the 'rag and bottle' method. In the USA, Ralph Waters, one of the country's few anaesthetic specialists, had been appointed to the University of Madigan in Wisconsin in 1927 and created a department distinguished by its close collaboration between practice and pharmacological and physiological sciences. His approach paid off and led to the development of a new anaesthetic, cyclopropane, and the introduction of the closed-circuit carbon dioxide absorption method. By the 1930s Waters's department was recognized as the 'Mecca of anaesthetics'. Waters was also noteworthy for his insistence that anaesthetists, rather than nurses, should administer anaesthetics. In Britain, the Second World War became the catalyst which drove the establishment of academic anaesthesia.

The Second World War was an international tragedy but the formation of the Emergency Medical Service and the need to train military doctors in anaesthetic administration set the foundations for the future. As press reports on Hitler's activities and Mussolini's campaigns began to grow, the focus turned to Oxford where Robert Macintosh, holder of the first chair of anaesthetics in the UK, headed an innovative team.

Golf may seem a curious inclusion in the history of anaesthesia. But it was a love of golf that brought the car manufacturer William Morris, later to become Lord Nuffield, and Robert Macintosh together in a symbiosis that embedded anaesthesia into academia. Morris had capitalized on the opportunities offered by motor cars in the 1900s and built up the Morris Motor Company in Cowley, Oxford. His success is legendary: by 1927 General Motors offered around £11 million for the business. Morris turned the offer down but in the same year purchased Huntercombe Golf Club near Henley to pursue his golfing activities. The club was the haunt of a handful of Guy's Hospital medics, one of whom was Robert Macintosh, then working in a dental anaesthetic cartel in Harley Street. Probably the only arrangement of its kind at the time, Macintosh and his two colleagues were supported by technicians who chauffeured them and their equipment between nursing homes and dental surgeries, and assisted them during anaesthetic administrations. Playing on the name of a local fuel supply company—The Mayfair Gas, Light, and Coke Company—the group was known as The Mayfair Gas, Fight, and Choke Company. Morris's long-established interest in medical matters was fuelled by dinner table discussions with the Guy's men. When Morris needed a minor operation in London, Macintosh administered the anaesthetic. Morris had undergone operations with anaesthesia before and found it to be a horrific experience. But on this occasion Morris's experience was different: he awoke asking why the operation had been delayed. Macintosh had put him to sleep with an injection of the recently developed Evipan.

The mask and inhalation with its feelings of suffocation was a thing of the past. Morris was deeply struck by the difference in experience from earlier anaesthetics. In 1936 he mentioned his plans to fund the establishment of a Postgraduate Medical School at Oxford with chairs in medicine, surgery, obstetrics, and gynaecology. Macintosh commented, 'I see they have forgotten anaesthetics again.' Morris, perhaps because he knew how much anaesthesia had changed recently, put pressure on the Oxford establishment and after many shenanigans Macintosh was appointed to a chair of anaesthetics: 'Then there was hell to pay,' recalled Macintosh. 'There was no-one at that time, no-one in the country, with the pretensions to fill a Chair in Anaesthetics. The highest science I knew was that ether was inflammable.'[242]

Macintosh's approach to his new task was pragmatic and direct. He agreed with his employers that most of 1937 would be devoted to study leave. Knowing he had never been formally trained in anaesthesia, he visited other departments, particularly Waters's department in Madison. Towards the end of 1937 Macintosh spent six weeks anaesthetizing for his friend Eastman Sheehan in the Spanish Civil War. The conditions of war meant cylinders of gas were unavailable. Macintosh returned to Oxford inspired to design a portable apparatus for volatile anaesthetic liquids that delivered a controllable and quantifiable dose and was easy to use. Thus the Oxford vaporizer was born. In many ways Macintosh's design was a descendant of Snow's early inhalers, built on the same principles though far more sophisticated. It meant, claimed the Nuffield Committee, that 'for the first time the vapour of any liquid anaesthetic can be administered in a known concentration, and this concentration can be varied at will.'[243] Macintosh capitalized on his links to Morris Motors and thousands of vaporizers were manufactured at Cowley between 1941 and 1947. Lord Nuffield presented supplies to the services during the Second World War. It was not the first time Macintosh had utilized the plant's skills. During the 1937 polio epidemic in Britain when there was a shortage of iron lung ventilators—the only treatment for the disease—Macintosh encouraged Morris to manufacture enough to supply every hospital in the country, promising him that lives would be saved.

By the time war broke out in September 1939, the Nuffield Department of Anaesthetics had established services for local hospitals and a research programme. Led by Macintosh, who became commodore in the Royal Air Force in 1941 with responsibility for anaesthetic services, Oxford was positioned to become a pivotal cog in the war effort. Macintosh toured RAF hospitals to review anaesthetic practice and found, as Guedel had during the First World War, that the lack of basic training and familiarity with equipment continued to impede practice. Only five regular medical officers in the army held the Diploma of Anaesthetics. Oxford responded with a twice-yearly refresher course for practitioners wishing to gain the Diploma. Each course attracted around forty-five or so attendants, including servicemen. Within a year or so, numbers of qualified anaesthetists doubled. In addition, the Oxford department pursued a wide-ranging research programme tackling wartime issues such as maintaining a respirable atmosphere in submarines; the maximum height for baling out from a plane without oxygen—it was reckoned to be 35,000 feet; the effects of the pressure from parachute harnesses on respiration during drops from high altitudes; and the design of life jackets. Anaesthetists continued to be willing volunteers. Edgar A. Pask, anaesthetist at the Royal Air Force Aviation Institute in Farnborough, was put under ether by Macintosh and then pushed into a swimming pool at Ealing studios to test new life-jacket designs—the problem being that current models turned their wearers face down in the water. Pask's diplomacy as much as his technological skills were put to the test when he was asked to devise a method whereby Winston Churchill could both breath oxygen and smoke his cigar during high-altitude flights: 'Our attempts were never successful,' Pask told Macintosh,

> the trouble was that the device worked unless you happened to put your tongue over the end of the cigar holder inside your mouth. This caused the oxygen to flow, not into Winston Churchill, but out past the incompetent non-return valve and through the lighted cigar. The wretched thing then burst into a bright white flame and about an inch of the best Havana disappeared before you could realise what had gone wrong.[244]

The war served to exemplify the benefits of specialist anaesthesia: 'Both Allies came to recognise as the war progressed, that, whereas a skilled experienced anaesthetist could "carry" an inexperienced surgeon, the reverse was catastrophic,' explained Philip Helliwell, who later became President of the Association of Anaesthetists.[245] The Japanese aircraft attack on the American fleet in Pearl Harbour in December 1941 produced around 3,400 casualties with many requiring surgery. Awful injuries coupled with difficult operating conditions prompted the use of Pentothal as the sole anaesthetic agent but the high mortality was later attributed to this decision. Such incidents served only to fuel anaesthetists' claims for widespread training and an academic base.

In 1908 the Society of Anaesthetists had amalgamated with the Royal Society of Medicine and became the Section of Anaesthetists. But the rules meant that the Section could only discuss academic issues, not undertake political activity. In 1923 the establishment of the *British Journal of Anaesthesia* provided a mouthpiece for professional concerns about low standards of practice and the poor status of anaesthetists. The founding of the Association of Anaesthetists by Birmingham anaesthetist Henry Featherborne in 1932 marked the beginning of a sustained effort to improve matters. In the aftermath of the war, the specialty benefited from the founding of the National Health Service, which established anaesthesia as one of the core functions in all hospital groups. Anaesthetists were quick to capitalize on the momentum of change. Until this point, the specialty's only academic qualification—the Diploma of Anaesthetics—was supervised by the Conjoint Board of the Royal Colleges of Physicians and Surgeons. A faculty of anaesthetists was set up within the Royal College of Surgeons in 1948 and gained seven hundred members in the first six months. By 1953 a Fellowship in Anaesthetics had been established and became the hallmark of specialist practice. The independent status of anaesthesia continued to grow, and in 1988, the College of Anaesthesia was founded, gaining a Royal Charter four years later.

Despite the incorporation of anaesthesia into the towers and spires of academia, problems continued to dog practice. From the 1920s regional anaesthesia—using nerve blocks to numb selected areas—and spinal anaesthesia made it possible to circumvent general anaesthesia in some cases. The range of anaesthetic agents had expanded with the introduction of cyclopropane and ethylene in the 1930s but like ether, these were inflammable. The burgeoning of electrically driven equipment in the operating theatre increased the risk of explosions. Concern grew. In 1930, Manchester anaesthetist K. B. Pinson estimated that at least 100 fires or explosions occurred each year. By 1944, a warning notice, drafted by a committee to investigate anaesthetic explosions, had been circulated to all operating theatres by the Ministry of Health. And, in 1956, the Ministry set up a working party on anaesthetic explosions, concluding that between 1947 and 1954 six million anaesthetics had been given using explosive agents; a total of thirty-six explosions had occurred and caused three deaths. The market for a new, non-toxic agent that combined volatility and anaesthetic potency with non-flammability was assured.

It was a close collaboration between a chemist, a pharmacist, and an anaesthetist that produced halothane, the first designer anaesthetic, at the Widnes Laboratory of ICI in the 1950s. A success story of considerable proportions, halothane was a fruit of ICI's postwar interest in pharmaceutical design, which had been marked by the establishment of a separate division in 1944. Since the 1930s, fluorine compounds had been developed at Widnes for use as refrigerants and aerosols—there had been an earlier suggestion that they may be potential anaesthetics. But in 1951, the idea of looking amongst the fluorine compounds for a volatile anaesthetic was raised again, this time by ICI's new research director of the General Chemicals Division, John Ferguson. In the 1930s Ferguson, then in ICI's Alkali Division, had searched for a volatile chemical that could be used as a fumigant to clear silos storing grain of destructive beetles. He noticed the chemical's narcotic effects on the beetles— they became unconscious and immobile but eventually recovered. Investigating further, he found that the chemical dosage required to produce narcosis was not proportionate to percentage by volume, but to the thermodynamic function known as thermodynamic activity, or relative saturation. Now, he took his work on narcosis to Charles Suckling, a young chemist working in the laboratory, and asked for his opinion. Suckling looked into the history of narcosis and, to everyone's surprise, discovered Ferguson's conclusions had been reached almost a century earlier by Snow. The search for a new anaesthetic began.

From the outset, the project was focused and holistic. Ferguson's understanding of narcosis provided a key to the enterprise as it enabled a good estimate to be made of the concentration of a given compound required to induce anaesthesia before submitting it to tests on animals. Suckling's knowledge of the chemistry of fluorinated compounds guided the selection of compounds for testing. He was also strongly influenced by a paper published in 1938 by M. H. Severs and Ralph Waters of Madison fame, which considered the criteria of the 'ideal' anaesthetic gas, and stressed the importance of accommodating the multiperspectives of patient, surgeon, anaesthetist, and manufacturer. An awareness of these different needs guided Suckling's work. It did not take long to strike gold. Halothane, the ninth compound tested, appeared promising. Suckling sent it to James Raventos, pharmacologist at ICI's pharmaceutical laboratories at Blackley, who he later described as 'wise, with an impish sense of humour and an infectious chuckle, cautious until sure of his facts'. Raventos was equally focused in his approach and had already developed a clear profile of the necessary pharmacological criteria. Through long and extensive animal experiments Raventos established halothane's distinctive pharmaceutical properties: nonflammable, non-toxic, high potency, rapid, uneventful induction and recovery. The first clinical trial was carried out at Manchester Royal Infirmary by anaesthetist Michael Johnstone, who had scrutinized Raventos's demonstrations of halothane on animals. Whilst a houseman, Johnstone had been instructed to administer the anaesthetic: 'drip the chloroform onto the mask ... if the patient turns grey call me,' he was told.[246] The patient did turn grey; the senior doctor did not know what to do. It was a life-changing moment for Johnstone, who subsequently chose to specialize in anaesthesia.

On 20 January 1956 Suckling received a telephone call from Raventos, who had been watching Johnstone at work: 'Halothane was used for the first time on human beings this morning in the Manchester Royal Infirmary with results which so far have proved entirely satisfactory,' Suckling reported to Ferguson and ICI management.[247] By September 1956 Johnstone reported around 500 successful administrations: 'after the first few cases it immediately became obvious that we were dealing with a drug totally different from all anaesthetics,' he said.[248] Clinical trials were extended to other centres and by the autumn of 1957, Fluothane (halothane's trade name) was on the world market. By 1958 many thousands of cases had been successfully anaesthetized with halothane with no deaths or postoperative illnesses in which the new agent was directly implicated. Things could have been very different: the first patient scheduled for the operating list on 20 January 1956 withdrew and awoke next morning with jaundice. Halothane might have been blamed for causing liver failure.

Critical in the success of halothane was the entrepreneurial contribution of the small firm Cyprane which, assisted by ICI, designed and marketed the 'Fluotec', a calibrated tap-controlled vaporizer which allowed second-by-second control of the low concentrations required in the clinical use of halothane. But in 1962, only months after revelations that thalidomide, introduced as a safe sleeping pill, had caused appalling foetal defects in the babies of around 5,000 women, a few cases of liver failure following halothane anaesthesia caused concern. The National Halothane Study was launched, led by John Bunker, Chairman of Stanford University's Department of Anaesthesia, and concluded in 1969 that liver damage was a potential but rare consequence of halothane anaesthesia. By this time, halothane had been used in the first human heart transplant performed by Dr Christiaan Barnard in Cape Town in December 1967. In 1973 Suckling and Raventos were awarded Philadelphia's John Scott Prize for 'men and women who make useful inventions', following in the footsteps of Sir Alexander Fleming and Marie Curie. Halothane was a watershed in the history of anaesthetic agents, providing a solution to old problems of inflammability (ether) and toxicity (chloroform). It was as much a product of the post-war burgeoning of the pharmaceutical industry as the individuals who created it, and the anaesthetists who built new standards of efficacy and safety on its chemical parameters. Still widely used in Third World countries, halothane was eventually overtaken in Europe and the USA by new anaesthetics with even shorter induction and recovery times. In turn, these facilitated an expansion in day-case surgery. By 1994 more than 60 per cent of surgical procedures were performed this way in the USA; the UK is rapidly following suit.

Whilst halothane was being developed, changing patterns of childbirth created new opportunities in obstetric anaesthesia. From the 1930s, fuelled partly by concern about levels of maternal mortality, the National Birthday Trust Fund led a campaign to extend pain relief in childbirth. Women fared well in some hospitals. At Queen Charlotte's Hospital in London, it was claimed that by 1930 more than 90 per cent of women received pain relief. But most births happened at home, and as chloroform remained the preserve of doctors, women delivered by midwives laboured without pain relief. In 1933 Liverpool anaesthetist R. J. Minnitt developed a machine for the self-administration of gas and air (Entonox), which was later approved for use by midwives. Over the first decades of the National Health Service, the numbers of babies being born in hospital rose and consultant anaesthetists were contracted for designated obstetric sessions. Within a hospital setting, supported by specialist anaesthesia, epidurals became, and remain, a popular form of pain relief. During this period, anaesthetists were also developing novel methods of caring for patients which would eventually form the basis of intensive care units.

An epidemic of polio in Copenhagen in 1952 prompted Danish anaesthetist Bjorn Ibsen to pioneer a new method of ventilation. Patients were suffering from a form of polio which paralysed swallowing, as well as spinal reflexes, and conventional ventilators could not prevent the aspiration of secretions into the lungs. Ibsen's idea was to avoid the dangers of aspiration by performing a tracheostomy and connecting the tracheostomy tube to an anaesthetic breathing system. The lungs could then be ventilated by manual compression of the reservoir bag although this needed to be continued for twenty-four hours a day for between two and three months of treatment. The manpower implications were tremendous and so was the will to succeed. Danish medical and dental students worked in six-hour shifts, and at the height of the epidemic, seventy patients were being manually ventilated. The mortality rate dropped from around 80 to 25 per cent and the new method was taken up for patients suffering trauma, head injuries, and drug overdoses, as well as respiratory problems. Again the new demands placed by surgery on anaesthesia stimulated new techniques and technology. Mechanical ventilation coupled with rigorous observation of the patient's bodily systems—nervous system, respiration, circulation, digestion, and so on—became an integral part of open-heart surgery from the late 1960s onwards and laid the structures for intensive care units.

In the twenty-first century, most intensive care units are managed by anaesthetists, as indeed are chronic pain services. During the 1950s, approaches to chronic pain underwent a significant shift. Again, the exigency of war played a part. During the Second World War, John Bonica, a young army anaesthetist who financed his medical training with the profits of professional wrestling, supervised anaesthetic services in Madigan Army Hospital. Housing 7,770 beds, the hospital admitted huge numbers of patients, many suffering pain after amputations or nerve injuries. In many cases, Bonica struggled to alleviate the patients' pain and looked to colleagues for help, sharing observations and ideas during weekly meetings. It was the beginning of a new, multidisciplinary approach to pain management that drew on a range of medical specialties—neurosurgery, neurology, psychiatry. 'The proper management of pain remains, after all, the most important obligation, the main objective, and the crowning achievement of *every* physician,' Bonica wrote in his definitive work, *The Management of Pain* (1953). He later established a Pain Centre at the University of Washington using the multidisciplinary approach and in 1974 founded the International Association for the Study of Pain. Pain clinics for chronic sufferers are now part and parcel of everyday medicine. Not all patients will find relief but the right to seek alleviation of chronic pain is never questioned. Residues of religious and moral opposition to pain relief had dissipated during the first half of the twentieth century: 'the use of anaesthetics is morally permissible ... the patient desirous of avoiding or of soothing the pain can, without disquiet of conscience, make use of the means discovered by science ... the Christian's duty of renunciation and of interior purification is not an obstacle to the use of anaesthetics,' affirmed the head of the Roman Catholic church, Pope Pius XII, in February 1957.[249]

Through the first part of the twentieth century, physical pain remained a problem for the dying; medical reluctance to prescribe too much opium persisted. Cicely Saunders, founder of our modern hospice movement, studied 900 patients at St Joseph's Hospice in 1964, and met patients who recounted tales of great suffering: 'The pain in the other hospital was so bad that if anyone came into the room, I would scream: "Don't touch me! Don't come near me!" ', one patient told Saunders.[250] Saunders's regimen of regular doses of opiates proved highly effective at preventing pain. Like William Munk before her, she argued that ideas of addiction were a myth for terminally ill patients. Saunders pioneered holistic care—though pain was pivotal, attention should also be given to the psychological stresses of terminal illness and family needs. In 1967 she founded St Christopher's Hospice, which admitted fifty-four in-patients during

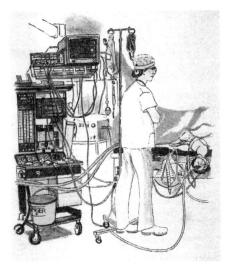

Figure 15 Today's anaesthetist flanked by anaesthetic technology, Chelsea and Westminster Hospital, 1996.

its first year and led the way for similar ventures. In the twenty-first century, palliative care is pretty successful in relieving the pains of death, though moral debates on the principles of euthanasia persist.

The world of today's anaesthesia seems separate and distinct from its early beginnings with ether and chloroform. The needle has replaced the mask and anaesthetists combine a raft of drugs with different functions—analgesia, amnesia, muscle relaxants, sedation, and so on—to create balanced anaesthesia. The proportion of daycase surgery increases year on year, as does the number of procedures performed under local anaesthesia. Since the 1980s, even the requirement for the anaesthetist to keep his finger on the pulse has disappeared, replaced by bleeping and flashing monitors.

New agents and new methods have greatly reduced the risks of anaesthetic fatalities to around 1 per 100,000 anaesthetics. At the Chelsea and Westminster Hospital in London, Professor Mervyn Maze and his team established the Eagle Simulator in 2000, a virtual operating theatre for training in anaesthesia and critical care.

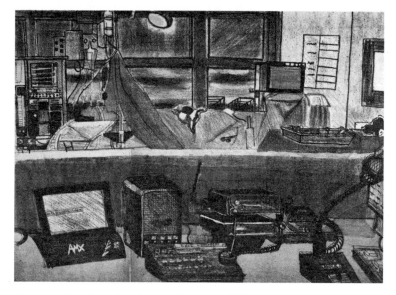

Figure 16 The Eagle Simulator at Chelsea and Westminster Hospital, a virtual operating theatre for training students in anaesthesia, 2000.

Some unpleasantries remain. Interruptions in the anaesthetic supply cause awareness in around 0.2 per cent of administrations. One to two million UK patients a year suffer from post-anaesthetic vomiting. It was, reported the Audit Commission in 1997, the most common cause for unplanned overnight hospitalization of day-case surgery patients. There are economic consequences for health services of course, as well as misery for patients. (Patients would opt for a small residue of pain rather than experience nausea and vomiting, suggests one study.) But the element that binds anaesthesia most tightly to its 1840s origins is the absence of definitive explanations in matters of mechanism and process.

Though we know much about the brain structures affected by anaesthesia, we do not know which are critical for anaesthesia; we know how cellular processes and molecules are modulated by anaesthesia, but cannot tell which of the modifications are key. To answer such questions requires, in part, more knowledge than we have about the relationship between neural and mental states, especially the states of consciousness and unconsciousness. The scientific frameworks into which we place anaesthesia have expanded dramatically since the late 1840s. The process of unconsciousness has become the focus of a raft of sciences including neurobiology and neurophysiology, as well as philosophy, psychology, and the comparatively new discipline of cognitive science. But explanations of what happens to the mind during unconsciousness remain elusive. Patients due to undergo anaesthesia are, perhaps, fearful, not so much because of its known risks, but because the nature of the process is unresolved. We ask the same question as did the first patients to breathe ether and chloroform: what will happen to our mind as our consciousness closes down? Few satisfying answers can be found, only contrasting accounts of individual experience. The journey into the shadowy terrains of unconsciousness and its landscape remains deeply personal and hard to characterize. For this reason, perhaps, the practice of anaesthesia is as much an art as a science. Some places have literally looked to art to alleviate pre-anaesthetic anxiety. The Chelsea Hospital for Women commissioned a ceiling mural for the anaesthetic room in 1959, hoping it would calm patients in the moments prior to induction. As patients, our safety depends on the anaesthetist's scientific and technological competence. But our emotional well being hinges more on a reassuring smile, or touch, as we embark on a journey into, as yet, unknown territories. Let the last word go to poet and physician at the University of California, David Watts, whose words capture the shared vulnerability of patient and anaesthetist as the voyage begins.

STARTING THE IV: ANESTHESIA
I am good at this.
The arm bends out, the vein
lies stretched and succulent,
transparent under the sheen
of alcohol. My fingers slide
the slippery skin, tracing
engorgement.

He says he's fine
but I see the cinch
of his muscles. So I tell him
I'm the best
and he eases,
slightly.

The needle glides
under the skin, beveled tip
in its slip along the vein
where I rest it
and let him relax. It waits
like a mosquito attached
by its sucker.

I press the tip
against the bulbous channel
and the wall bends, resisting
for an instant, then,
as if capitulating, gives way
and a column of blood
enters the tubing.

I have learned not to hesitate here,
not to let fears of my own
about anesthesia, about loss
of control, get in the way.
He will want to descend
quickly, not pausing
to feel each station of detachment.
I take the control he gives me
and bring him down.

ENDNOTES

CHAPTER I: INTRODUCTION

1. Fanny Burney, *Selected Letters and Journals*, ed. Joyce Hemlow (Oxford: Oxford University Press, 1986), 127–41.
2. Quoted in Claire Tomalin, *Samuel Pepys: The Unequalled Self* (London: Viking, 2002), 61.
3. Quoted in Peter Stanley, *For Fear of Pain, British Surgery 1790–1850* (Amsterdam and New York: Rodopi, 2003), 204–5.
4. Quoted in W. F. Bynum, *Science and the Practice of Medicine in the Nineteenth Century* (Cambridge: Cambridge University Press, 1993), 17.
5. Quoted in Roy Porter and Dorothy Porter, *In Sickness and In Health: The English Experience 1650-1850* (London: Fourth Estate, 1988), 70.
6. David Hume, *Essays and Treatises on Several Subjects* (Edinburgh: Bell and Bradfute, 1825), 6–7.
7. Quoted in Jenny Uglow, *The Lunar Men: The Friends Who Made the Future* (London: Faber and Faber, 2002), 231.
8. Ibid. 442.
9. Quoted in Roy Porter, *Flesh in the Age of Reason* (London: Allen Lane, 2003), 415.
10. Humphry Davy, *Researches, Chemical and Philosophical; Chiefly Concerning Nitrous Oxide, or Dephlogisticated Nitrous Air and its Respiration* (London: Butterworths, 1972), 453–96.
11. Quoted in A. Hayter, *Opium and the Romantic Imagination* (London: Faber and Faber, 1971), 75.
12. Davy, *Researches, Chemical and Philosophical*, 519.

13. Ibid. 499.
14. Ibid. 518.
15. Ibid. 558.
16. Letter from Henry Hill Hickman to Thomas Andrew Knight, 21 February 1824, held at the Wellcome Trust Library, London.
17. Quoted in W. D. A. Smith, *Henry Hill Hickman* (Sheffield: History of Anaesthesia Society, 2005), 31.
18. Ibid.
19. Reprinted in W. D. A. Smith, *Under the Influence* (Macmillan: London, 1982), 34.
20. Ibid. 35.
21. Quoted in Richard J. Wolfe, *Tarnished Idol, William Thomas Green Morton and the Introduction of Surgical Anaesthesia, A Chronicle of the Ether Controversy* (San Anselmo, CA: Norman Publishing, 2001), 51–2.
22. Quoted in Martin S. Pernick, *A Calculus of Suffering: Pain, Professionalism and Anaesthesia in Nineteenth Century America* (New York: Columbia University Press, 1985), 72.
23. Quoted in Stanley, *For Fear of Pain*, 288.
24. *Lancet* I (1843–4), 500.
25. Wolfe, *Tarnished Idol*, 145.
26. Ibid. 67.
27. Ibid. 69.
28. *Lancet* I (1847), 6–8.
29. Quoted in Barbara M. Duncum, *The Development of Inhalation Anaesthesia* (London: Royal Society of Medicine Press, 1994), 122.

CHAPTER 2: DISCOVERIES

30. James Robinson, *On the Inhalation of the Vapour of Ether*, with a preface by Richard H. Ellis (Eastbourne: Balliere Tindall, 1983), 1.
31. Ibid. 6.
32. Ibid.
33. Quoted in Barbara M. Duncum, *The Development of Inhalation Anaesthesia* (London: Royal Society of Medicine Press, 1994), 562.

34. Quoted in Roselyne Rey, *The History of Pain*, trans. Louise Elliott Wallace, J. A. Cadden, and S. W. Cadden (Cambridge, MA: Harvard University Press, 1995), 157.
35. Quoted in Thomas Dormandy, *The Worst of Evils* (New Haven and London: Yale University Press, 2006), 235.
36. *London Medical Gazette* 38 (1846), 1089.
37. Robinson, *On the Inhalation of the Vapour of Ether*, 20-1.
38. Ibid. 27.
39. Ibid. 43.
40. Quoted in Duncum, *The Development of Inhalation Anaesthesia*, 153.
41. *London Medical Gazette* 31 (1842–3), 813.
42. *Lancet* I (1847), 99–100.
43. Ibid. 120–1.
44. John Snow, *On the Inhalation of Ether in Surgical Operations* (London: Churchill, 1847), 21.
45. John Snow, *On Chloroform and Other Anaesthetics* (London: Churchill, 1858), p. xiv.
46. *London Medical Gazette* 39 (1847), 500.
47. *Lancet* I (1847), 343.
48. Quoted in Dormandy, *The Worst of Evils*, 237.
49. *Lancet* I (1847), 551–4.
50. Snow, *On Ether*, 5 and 33.
51. Quoted in Manfred Waserman, 'Sir James Y. Simpson and London's "Conservative and So Curiously Prejudiced" Dr Ramsbotham', *British Medical Journal* 2 (1980), 158–61.
52. Quoted in David Wilkinson, 'A Strange Little Book', *Anaesthesia* 58 (2003), 36–41.
53. *Lancet* II (1847), 575–6.
54. K. Bryn Thomas, 'Chloroform at Christmas', *Anaesthesia* 30 (1975), 219–22.
55. *The Times*, 3 February 1848, 8.
56. Quoted in Stephanie J. Snow, *Operations without Pain: The Practice and Science of Anaesthesia in Victorian Britain* (London: Palgrave Macmillan, 2006), 84.
57. *London Medical Gazette* 6 (1848), 277–8.
58. Snow, *On Chloroform*, p. xiv.

59. Quoted in Duncum, *The Development of Inhalation Anaesthesia*, 204–6.
60. *Lancet* II (1872), 241–2.

CHAPTER 3: ANAESTHESIA IN ACTION

61. Quoted in Juliet Barker, *The Brontes* (London: Weidenfeld and Nicolson, 1994), 519.
62. Quoted in Martin S. Pernick, *A Calculus of Suffering: Pain, Professionalism and Anaesthesia in Nineteenth Century America* (New York: Columbia University Press, 1985), 36.
63. Quoted in Stephanie J. Snow, *Operations without Pain: The Practice and Science of Anaesthesia in Victorian Britain* (London: Palgrave Macmillan, 2006), 131.
64. Quoted in Pernick, *A Calculus of Suffering*, 36.
65. Quoted in Snow, *Operations without Pain*, 72.
66. Quoted in Thomas Dormandy, *The Worst of Evils* (New Haven and London: Yale University Press, 2006), 236.
67. *London Medical Gazette* 8 (1849), 455.
68. James Robinson, *On the Inhalation of the Vapour of Ether*, with a preface by Richard H. Ellis (Eastbourne: Balliere Tindall, 1983), 37.
69. Quoted in Barker, *The Brontes*, 934.
70. Quoted in Dormandy, *The Worst of Evils*, 236.
71. Quoted in Roselyne Rey, *The History of Pain*, trans. Louise Elliott Wallace, J. A. Cadden, and S. W. Cadden (Cambridge, MA: Harvard University Press, 1995), 163.
72. Quoted in Peter Stanley, *For Fear of Pain, British Surgery 1790–1850* (Amsterdam–New York: Rodopi, 2003), 299.
73. James Miller, *Principles of Surgery* (Edinburgh, 1846), 5.
74. *Lancet* I (1847), 553.
75. Quoted in Stanley, *For Fear of Pain*, 300.
76. Quoted in Pernick, *A Calculus of Suffering*, 48.
77. *Lancet* II (1854), 513.
78. Quoted in Douglas Hurd, *Robert Peel: A Biography* (London: Weidenfeld and Nicolson, 2007), 386.
79. Quoted in Snow, *Operations without Pain*, 100.

80. C. J. B. Williams, *Principles of Medicine*, 6th edn (1843), 26.
81. Sarah Stickney Ellis, *The Women of England, Their Social Duties and Domestic Habits* (London: Fisher, Son & Co., 1839).
82. Sarah Stickney Ellis, *The Wives of England, Their Relative Duties, Domestic Influence, and Social Obligations* (London: Fisher, Son & Co., 1843).
83. J. Roberton, *Essays and Notes on the Physiology and Diseases of Women* (London, 1851), 1–2.
84. Quoted in Pernick, *A Calculus of Suffering*, 149.
85. Ibid. 174.
86. Ibid. 173.
87. Ibid. 175.
88. John Snow, *On Chloroform and Other Anaesthetics* (London: Churchill, 1858), 52.
89. Quoted in Pernick, *A Calculus of Suffering*, 176.
90. Quoted in Dormandy, *The Worst of Evils*, 290.
91. Quoted in Pernick, *A Calculus of Suffering*, 154.
92. James Young Simpson, *Anaesthesia or the Employment of Chloroform and Ether in Surgery, Midwifery etc.* (Philadelphia: Lindsay and Blakiston, 1849), 246.
93. *Lancet* II (1841–2), 404.
94. Quoted in H. Marcus Bird, 'James Arnott, M.D.: A Pioneer in Refrigeration Analgesia', *Anaesthesia* 4 (1949), 10–17.
95. *Lancet* I (1850), 283.
96. Richard H. Ellis, *The Casebooks of Dr John Snow* (*Medical History*, Suppl. 14, London, 1994), 28 April 1852.
97. Ibid. 30 April 1850.
98. Ibid. 2 April 1853.
9.9 Ibid. 11 August 1852.
100. Ibid. 30 June 1849.
101. Ibid. 25 July 1849.

CHAPTER 4: WOMEN, SEX, AND SUFFERING

102. Edward Wagenknecht, *Mrs Longfellow: Selected Letters and Journals* (London: P. Owen, 1959), 129–30.

103. S. W. J. Merriman, *Arguments against the Indiscriminate Use of Chloroform in Midwifery* (London: John Churchill, 1848), 24.
104. *Lancet* I (1847), 377.
105. Quoted in Stephanie J. Snow, *Operations without Pain: The Practice and Science of Anaesthesia in Victorian Britain* (London: Palgrave Macmillan, 2006), 77.
106. Quoted in Martin S. Pernick, *A Calculus of Suffering: Pain, Professionalism and Anaesthesia in Nineteenth Century America* (New York: Columbia University Press, 1985), 103.
107. George Gream, *Remarks on the Employment of Anaesthetic Agents in Midwifery* (London: John Churchill, 1848), 7.
108. *Lancet* I (1848), 97–8.
109. Quoted in Linda Stratmann, *Chloroform: The Quest for Oblivion* (Stroud: Sutton Publishing, 2003), 44.
110. Quoted in Janet Browne, *Charles Darwin, Voyaging* (Princeton, NJ: Princeton University Press, 1995), 44.
111. All references can be found on the University of Cambridge Charles Darwin correspondence site, accessed 31 December 2007: http://www.darwinproject.ac.uk.
112. Graham Storey and K. J. Fielding, *The Letters of Charles Dickens*, vol. 5: *1847–1849* (Oxford: Clarendon Press, 1981), 486–7.
113. Roger Fulford (ed.), *Dearest Child: Letters between Queen Victoria and the Princess Royal, 1858–61* (London: Evans Brothers, 1964), 195, 162; Elizabeth Longford, *Victoria RI* (London: Weidenfeld and Nicolson, 1964), 154
114. Longford, *Victoria RI*, 94–105
115. John Snow, *On Chloroform and Other Anaesthetics* (London: Churchill, 1858), p. xxxv.
116. Richard H. Ellis, *The Casebooks of Dr John Snow* (*Medical History*, Suppl. 14, London, 1994), 7 April 1853.
117. *Association Medical Journal* (1853), 500–2.
118. Snow, *On Chloroform*, p. xxxi.
119. *Association Medical Journal* (1853), 318.
120. *Lancet* I (1853), 453.
121. *Medical Times and Gazette* 6 (1853), 526–7.
122. *Association Medical Journal* (1853), 450.

123. Ibid. 575.
124. Ellis, 23 April 1853.
125. Ibid. 28 April 1853.
126. Ibid. 7 April 1857.
127. Longford, *Victoria RI*, 261 and 265.
128. Ellis, 14 April 1857.
129. Longford, *Victoria RI*, 266.
130. *Lancet* I (1857), 410.
131. Hannah Pakula, *An Uncommon Woman—The Empress Frederick: Daughter of Queen Victoria, Wife of the Crown Prince of Prussia, Mother of Kaiser Wilhelm* (Simon and Schuster, 1995), 137.

CHAPTER 5: ON BATTLEFIELDS

132. John Raymond (ed.), *Queen Victoria's Early Letters* (London: B. T. Batsford, 1963), 198.
133. Quoted in Alexis Troubetzkoy, *The Crimean War* (London: Constable and Robinson, 2006), pp. xv, 210.
134. Quoted in ibid. 38.
135. *Lancet* II (1856), 3.
136. Quoted in Henry Connor, 'The Use of Chloroform by British Army Surgeons during the Crimean War', *Medical History* 42 (1998), 161–93, esp. 163.
137. *Lancet* I (1847), 551–4.
138. *Lancet* I (1855), 196.
139. *Lancet* II (1848), 5.
140. Quoted in Linda Stratmann, *Chloroform: The Quest for Oblivion* (Stroud: Sutton Publishing, 2003), 97.
141. *Lancet* I (1851), 96.
142. *The Times*, 12 October 1854, 9.
143. *Monthly Journal of Medical Science* 19 (1854), 475–6.
144. *Lancet* II (1856), 79.
145. Quoted in *National Army Museum Online: Exhibitions: The Victoria Cross: VC Heroes: Mark Walker VC*. Accessed 31 December 2007. Available at URL: http://www.national-army-museum.ac.uk/exhibitions/vc/page4.shtml.

146. Quoted in Connor, 'The Use of Chloroform', 177.
147. *Lancet* I (1855), 648.
148. *Lancet* II (1854), 389.
149. Ibid. 495.
150. *Medical Times and Gazette* II (1854), 604.
151. Ibid. 664–5.
152. *The Times*, 12 October 1854, 7; and 13 October 1854, 8.
153. Quoted in Sue M. Goldie (ed.), *'I Have Done My Duty': Florence Nightingale in the Crimean War 1854–56* (Iowa City, IA: University of Iowa Press, 1987), 24.
154. Ibid. 36-8.
155. *Lancet* II (1899), 207.
156. *Lancet* I (1855), 582.
157. *Lancet* I (1856), 650.
158. *Monthly Journal of Medicine* 20 (1855), 434.
159. Quoted in Troubetzkoy, *The Crimean War*, 280–1.
160. Quoted in Stratmann, *Chloroform*, 102.
161. George Guthrie, *Commentaries on the Surgery of the War etc.*, 6th edn (London: John Churchill, 1855), 618.
162. *Lancet* II (1855), 361.
163. J. Julian Chisholm, *A Manual of Military Surgery for the Use of Surgeons of the Confederate States Army* (Columbia: Evans and Cogswell, 1864), 427.
164. Quoted in Stratmann, *Chloroform*, 106.
165. William Williams Keen, *Addresses and Other Papers [on medicine]*, (Philadelphia and London: W. B. Saunders & Co., 1905).
166. Quoted in Hilaire McCoubrey, 'Before Geneva Law: A British Surgeon in the Crimean War', *International Review of the Red Cross*, no. 304 (1995), 69–80.
167. *Lancet* I (1847), 551–4.
168. Quoted in Henry Connor, 'The Use of Anaesthesia to Diagnose Malingering in the 19th Century', *Journal of the Royal Society of Medicine* 9 (1999), 457.
169. Quoted in Thomas Trotter, *A View of the Nervous Temperament* (London: Longman, 1807).
170. Quoted in Stratmann, *Chloroform*, 108.

171. Chisolm, *A Manual of Military Surgery*, 380–1.

172. Louisa May Alcott, *Sketches of Hospital Practice* (Boston: James Redpath, 1863), 96–8.

CHAPTER 6: THE DARK SIDE OF CHLOROFORM

173. *The Times*, 5 October 1849, 3.

174. John Snow, *Letter to the Right Honourable Lord Campbell, Lord Chief Justice of the Course of Queen's Bench, on the Clause Respecting Chloroform in the Proposed Prevention of Offences Bill* (London: John Churchill, 1851), 9–11.

175. Ibid. 4.

176. *Household Words* 7 (1851), 151–5.

177. *The Times*, 1 May 1850, 8.

178. *Lancet* II (1865), 490.

179. *The Times*, 3 December 1875, 5.

180. *Lancet* I (1886), 968–70, 1017–18.

181. Quoted in R. J. Flanagan and K. D. Watson, 'Chloroform— Murder or Suicide: Sir Thomas Stevenson and His Role in the Trial of Adelaide Bartlett', *History of Anaesthesia Proceedings* 32 (2003), 40–9.

182. Sir John Hall (ed.), *Trial of Adelaide Bartlett* (Edinburgh and London: William Hodge & Co., 1927).

183. Ibid.

184. *The Times*, 5 November 1847, 3.

185. Quoted in Ornella Moscucci, *The Science of Woman: Gynaecology and Gender in England, 1800–1929* (Cambridge: Cambridge University Press, 1990), 112–17.

186. Quoted in Richard Ellmann, *Oscar Wilde* (London: Hamish Hamilton, 1987), 15.

187. *Lancet* II (1864), 720–1.

188. Ellmann, *Oscar Wilde*, 15.

189. D. W. Buxton, *Anaesthetics, Their Uses and Administration* (London: H. K. Lewis, 1888), 149–50.

190. *Anaesthesia* 46 (1991), 328–9

191. Quoted in Linda Stratmann, *Chloroform: The Quest for Oblivion* (Stroud: Sutton Publishing, 2003), 134.
192. Quoted in Frederick Whyte, *The Life of W. T. Stead,* 2 vols. (London: Johnathan Cape, 1925), i. 304–6.
193. *Lancet* II (1855), 905, 972–3.
194. *Household Words* 7 (1853), 181.
195. Frederick Treves, 'Anaesthetics in Operative Surgery', *Practitioner* 57 (1896), 377–83.

CHAPTER 7: CHANGED UNDERSTANDINGS OF PAIN

196. *The Times*, 27 May 1868, 9.
197. *Lancet* I (1862), 345–7.
198. *Lancet* I (1871), 641–2, 679–80, 739–41, 816–17.
199. *Lancet* I (1888), 21–2.
200. William Munk, *Euthanasia: or Medical Treatment in Aid of an Easy Death* (London, 1887), 22–6.
201. Leon Edel (ed.), *The Diary of Alice James* (Boston: Northeastern University Press, 1999), 15.
202. Quoted in Laura Davidow Hirshbein, 'William Osler and *The Fixed Period*: Conflicting Medical and Popular Ideas about Old Age', *Archives of Internal Medicine* 161 (2001), 2074–8.
203. Quoted in Victoria Glendinning, *Trollope* (Pimlico, 1993), 497.
204. Quoted in Roy Porter, *The Greatest Benefit to Mankind: A Medical History of Humanity* (New York: W. W. Norton, 1997), 386.
205. *Lancet* II (1887), 391.
206. Harriet Martineau, *Life in the Sick-Room* (London: Edward Moxon, 1844).
207. Quoted in Adrian Desmond and James Moore, *Darwin* (London: Penguin, 1992), 427–8.
208. Quoted in Janet Browne, *Charles Darwin, The Power of Place* (London; Pimlico, 2003), 421.
209. Letter from Christina Rossetti to Dante Gabriel Rossetti, 10 September 1875. Accessed 31 December 2007. Available at URL: http://rotunda.upress.virginia.edu:8080/crossetti/.
210. *The Times*, 18 April 1881, 10.

211. Ibid. 19 April 1881, 8.
212. *Lancet* I (1840), 336.
213. Letter from Christina Rossetti to William Michael Rossetti, July 1889. Accessed 31 December 2007. Available at URL: http://rotunda.upress.virginia.edu.8080/crossetti/. The so-called 'operation' was most probably inoculation against rabies. Louis Pasteur had developed an antirabies vaccine in 1884 and in 1888 opened the Pasteur Institute.
214. Quoted in Martin J. Wiener, *Reconstructing the Criminal: Culture, Law and Policy in England, 1830–1914* (Cambridge: Cambridge University Press, 1994), 96.
215. *The Times*, 14 November 1849, 4.
216. Ibid. 14 August 1868, 10.
217. Ibid. 17 December 1894, 9.
218. Quoted in Wiener *Reconstructing the Criminal*, 334.
219. William James, *The Varieties of Religious Experience* (New York, 1902), 239.
220. Quoted in Browne, *Charles Darwin*, 502.
221. Charles Voysey, *The Mystery of Pain, Death and Sin, and Discourses in Refutation of Atheism* (London and Edinburgh, 1878).
222. Quoted in Robin Gilmour, *The Victorian Period: The Intellectual and Cultural Context of English Literature, 1830–1890* (London: Longmans, 1993), 87.
223. John C. Broderick et al. (eds), *Henry D. Thoreau: Journal*, vol. 3: *1848–1851* (Princeton: Princeton University Press, 1990), 218.
224. Quoted in James, *Varieties of Religious Experience*, 302.
225. Ibid.
226. Guy de Maupassant, *Afloat* (London: Peter Owen, 1995), 72–3.

CHAPTER 8: INTO THE
TWENTIETH CENTURY AND BEYOND

227. *Lancet* I (1902), 1815.
228. *British Medical Journal* II (1900), 284–9.
229. Quoted in Ian A. Burney, *Bodies of Evidence* (Baltimore: Johns Hopkins University Press, 2000), 142.

230. Quoted in Barbara M. Duncum, *The Development of Inhalation Anaesthesia* (London: Royal Society of Medicine Press, 1994), 432.
231. Quoted in ibid. 454.
232. *The Times*, 24 June 1922, 5.
233. *British Medical Journal* I (1923), 996.
234. Quoted in Ralph Waters, 'Arthur E. Guedel', *British Journal of Anaesthesia* 24 (1952), 292–9.
235. Stanley Rowbotham, 'Ivan Magill', *British Journal of Anaesthesia* 23 (1951), 49–55.
236. Quoted in Keith Sykes, 'The Griffith Legacy', *Canadian Journal of Anaesthesia* 40 (1993), 365–74.
237. *Lancet* I (1943), 478.
238. Ibid. 600.
239. *Lancet* II (1946), 80–4.
240. *British Medical Journal* I (1950), 247–8.
241. Keith Sykes and John Bunker, *Anaesthesia and the Practice of Medicine: Historical Perspectives* (London: Royal Society of Medicine Press, 2007).
242. Quoted in Jennifer Beinart, *A History of the Nuffield Department of Anaesthetics, Oxford 1937–1987* (Oxford: Oxford University Press, 1987), 27.
243. Ibid. 55.
244. Ibid. 51.
245. Ibid. 76.
246. Colin Suckling, 'Recollections and Reflections on the Discovery of Halothane', presented to the 6th International Symposium on the History of Anaesthesia, Queens College, Cambridge, 17 September 2005.
247. Interview with Charles Suckling, May 2007.
248. Michael Johnstone, 'The Clinical Trial', *Manchester University Medical School Gazette* 37 (1958), 60.
249. *The Times*, 25 February 1957, 6.
250. Quoted in Thomas Dormandy, *The Worst of Evils* (New Haven and London: Yale University Press, 2006), 495.

FURTHER READING

For those wishing to learn more about the history of medicine and indeed, anaesthesia, I list below some general reading and the sources I have drawn on most heavily. Any historical work is dependent upon a raft of other scholarship and this book is no exception. The in-depth historiographical framework upon which this book is based is laid out in my earlier work— *Operations without Pain: The Practice and Science of Anaesthesia in Victorian Britain* (Palgrave Macmillan, 2006). For this reason, here I have mostly omitted scholarly articles because they are less accessible to the general reader.

HISTORY OF MEDICINE

John C. Burnham, *What is Medical History?* (Cambridge: Polity Press, 2005).

W. F. Bynum, *Science and the Practice of Medicine in the Nineteenth Century* (Cambridge: Cambridge University Press, 1993).

—— and Roy Porter (eds), *Companion Encyclopaedia of the History of Medicine*, 2 vols (London and New York: Routledge, 1993).

—— et al., *The Western Medical Tradition, 1800-2000* (Cambridge: Cambridge University Press, 2006).

Roger Cooter and J. V. Pickstone (eds), *Companion to Medicine in the Twentieth Century* (London and New York: Routledge, 2003).

Anne Digby, *Making a Medical Living: Doctors and Patients in the English Market for Medicine, 1720–1911* (Cambridge: Cambridge University Press, 1994).

Joan Lane, *A Social History of Medicine: Health, Healing and Disease in England, 1750-1950* (London: Routledge, 2001).

J. V. Pickstone, *Ways of Knowing, A New History of Science, Technology and Medicine* (Manchester: Manchester University Press, 2000).

Roy Porter, *The Greatest Benefit to Mankind: A Medical History of Humanity* (New York: W. W. Norton, 1997).

HISTORY OF ANAESTHESIA

Richard S. Atkinson and Thomas B. Boulton, *The History of Anaesthesia* (London: Royal Society of Medicine Services, 1989).

A. Barr et al. (eds), *Essays on the History of Anaesthesia* (London: Royal Society of Medicine Press, 1996).

Norman A. Bergman, *The Genesis of Surgical Anaesthesia* (Park Ridge, IL: Wood Library, Museum of Anesthesiology, 1998).

F. F. Cartwright, *English Pioneers of Anaesthesia* (Bristol and London: John Wright, 1952).

Thomas Dormandy, *The Worst of Evils* (New Haven and London: Yale University Press, 2006).

Barbara M. Duncum, *The Development of Inhalation Anaesthesia* (London: Royal Society of Medicine Press, 1994).

Richard H. Ellis, *The Casebooks of Dr John Snow* (*Medical History*, Suppl. 14, London, 1994).

Thomas E. Keys, *The History of Surgical Anaesthesia* (New York: Schumans, 1945).

Christopher Lawrence and Ghislaine Lawrence, *No Laughing Matter: Historical Aspects of Anaesthesia* (London: Wellcome Institute for the History of Medicine, 1987).

J. Roger Maltby, *Notable Names in Anaesthesia* (London: Royal Society of Medicine Press, 2002).

Martin S. Pernick, *A Calculus of Suffering: Pain, Professionalism and Anaesthesia in Nineteenth Century America* (New York: Columbia University Press, 1985).

G. B. Rushman et al., *A Short History of Anaesthesia: The First 150 Years* (London: Butterworth Heinemann, 1996).

W. D. A. Smith, *Under the Influence* (Macmillan: London, 1982).

——, *Henry Hill Hickman* (Sheffield: History of Anaesthesia Society, 2005).

Linda Stratmann, *Chloroform: The Quest for Oblivion* (Stroud: Sutton Publishing, 2003).

Keith Sykes and John Bunker, *Anaesthesia and the Practice of Medicine: Historical Perspectives* (London: Royal Society of Medicine Press, 2007).

W. S. Sykes, *Essays on the First Hundred Years of Anaesthesia*, 3 vols. (Edinburgh: Livingstone, 1960, 1961, 1982).

Richard J. Wolfe, *Tarnished Idol, William Thomas Green Morton and the Introduction of Surgical Anaesthesia, A Chronicle of the Ether Controversy* (San Anselmo, CA: Norman Publishing, 2001).

CHAPTER 1: INTRODUCTION

Philippe Aries, *The Hour of Our Death* (Oxford: Oxford University Press, 1991).

Virginia Berridge and Griffith Edwards, *Opium and the People* (New Haven and London: Yale University Press, 1987).

Hilton Boyd, *The Age of Atonement: The Influence of Evangelicism on Social and Economic Thought, 1795–1865* (Oxford: Clarendon Press, 1988).

A. S. Byatt, *Unruly Times: Wordsworth and Coleridge in Their Time* (London: Vintage, 1997).

W. F. Bynum and Roy Porter (eds), *William Hunter and the Eighteenth-Century Medical World* (Cambridge: Cambridge University Press, 1985).

Michael Crumplin, *Men of Steel: Surgery in the Napoleonic Wars* (London: Quiller Press, 2007).

J. Golinski, *Science as Public Culture: Chemistry and Enlightenment in Britain, 1760–1820* (Cambridge: Cambridge University Press, 1992).

A. Hayter, *Opium and the Romantic Imagination* (London: Faber and Faber, 1971).

Christine Hillam (ed.), *Dental Practice in Europe at the End of the 18th Century* (Amsterdam and New York: Rodopi, 2003).

David Knight, *Humphry Davy* (Oxford: Blackwell, 1992).

Roy Porter, *The Enlightenment* (Hampshire: Macmillan, 1990).

———, *Doctor of Society* (London and New York: Routledge, 1992).

———, *Flesh in the Age of Reason* (London: Allen Lane, 2003).

Roselyne Rey, *The History of Pain*, trans. Louise Elliott Wallace, J. A.
Cadden, and S. W. Cadden (Cambridge, MA: Harvard University
Press, 1995).

Peter Stanley, *For Fear of Pain, British Surgery 1790–1850* (Amsterdam–
New York: Rodopi, 2003).

Jenny Uglow, *The Lunar Men: The Friends Who Made the Future*
(London: Faber and Faber, 2002).

Alison Winter, *Mesmerized: Powers of Mind in Victorian Britain* (Chicago:
University of Chicago Press, 1998).

CHAPTER 2: DISCOVERIES
CHAPTER 3: ANAESTHESIA IN ACTION

Richard S. Atkinson, *James Simpson and Chloroform* (London: Priory
Press, 1973).

F. F. Cartwright, *The Development of Modern Surgery* (New York: Barker,
1968).

Kenneth Allen De Ville, *Medical Malpractice in Nineteenth Century
America* (New York: New York University Press, 1990).

Martin S. Pernick, *A Calculus of Suffering: Pain, Professionalism and
Anaesthesia in Nineteenth Century America* (New York: Columbia
University Press, 1985).

J. A. Shepherd, *Simpson and Syme of Edinburgh* (Edinburgh: E and
S Livingstone, 1969).

Peter Vinten-Johansen et al., *Cholera, Chloroform and the Science of
Medicine, A Life of John Snow* (Oxford: Oxford University Press,
2003).

CHAPTER 4: WOMEN, SEX, AND SUFFERING

Peter Ackroyd, *Dickens* (London: Guild, 1990).

Janet Browne, *Charles Darwin, Voyaging* (Princeton, NJ: Princeton
University Press, 1995).

——, *Charles Darwin, The Power of Place* (London: Pimlico, 2003).

Donald Caton, *What a Blessing She Had Chloroform* (New Haven and
London: Yale University Press, 1999).

Roger Fulford (ed.), *Dearest Child: Letters between Queen Victoria and the Princess Royal, 1858–61* (London: Evans Brothers, 1964).

Judith W. Leavitt, *Brought to Bed: Childbearing in America 1750 to 1950* (Oxford: Oxford University Press, 1986).

Elizabeth Longford, *Victoria RI* (London: Weidenfeld and Nicolson, 1964).

Irvine Loudon, *Death in Childbirth: An International Study of Maternal Care and Maternal Mortality 1800–1950* (Oxford: Clarendon Press, 1992).

Ornella Moscucci, *The Science of Woman. Gynaecology and Gender in England, 1800–1929* (Cambridge: Cambridge University Press, 1990).

Mary Poovey, *Uneven Developments: The Ideological Work of Gender in Mid-Victorian England* (London: Virago, 1989).

John Raymond (ed.), *Queen Victoria's Early Letters* (London: B. T. Batsford, 1963).

Elaine Showalter, *The Female Malady, Women, Madness and English Culture, 1830–1980* (London: Virago, 1987).

Graham Storey and K. J. Fielding, *The Letters of Charles Dickens*, vol. 5: *1847–1849* (Oxford: Clarendon Press, 1981).

Dorothy Thompson, *Queen Victoria: Gender and Power* (London: Virago, 1990).

Martha Vicinus, *A Widening Sphere: Changing Roles of Victorian Women* (Bloomington, IN: Indiana University Press, 1977).

Edward Wagenknecht, *Mrs Longfellow: Selected Letters and Journals* (London: P. Owen, 1959).

CHAPTER 5: ON BATTLEFIELDS

Maurice S. Albin, 'The Use of Anesthetics during the Civil War, 1861–65', *Pharmacy in History* 42 (2000), 99–114.

Tim Coates (ed.), *Florence Nightingale and the Crimea, 1854–55* (London: The Stationery Office, 2000).

Henry Connor, 'The Use of Chloroform by British Army Surgeons during the Crimean War', *Medical History*, 42 (1998), 161–93.

Sue M. Goldie (ed.), *'I Have Done My Duty': Florence Nightingale in the Crimean War 1854–56* (Iowa City, IA: University of Iowa Press, 1987).

J. A. Shepherd, *The Crimean Doctors: A History of the British Medical Services in the Crimean War* (Liverpool: Liverpool University Press, 1991).

Alexis Troubetzkoy, *The Crimean War* (London: Constable and Robinson, 2006).

CHAPTER 6: THE DARK SIDE OF CHLOROFORM

Ian Burney, *Poison, Detection, and the Victorian Imagination* (Manchester and New York: Manchester University Press, 2006).

Richard Ellmann, *Oscar Wilde* (London: Hamish Hamilton, 1987).

Frank Mort, *Dangerous Sexualities: Medico-Moral Politics in England since 1830* (London and New York: Routledge, 2000).

A. N. Wilson, *The Victorians* (London: Arrow Books, 2003).

CHAPTER 7: CHANGED UNDERSTANDINGS OF PAIN

Lucy Bending, *The Representation of Bodily Pain in Late Nineteenth-Century English Culture* (Oxford: Oxford University Press, 2000).

Roger French, *Antivivisection and Medical Science in Victorian Society* (Princeton, NJ: Princeton University Press, 1975).

David Garland, *Punishment and Welfare: A History of Penal Strategies* (Aldershot: Gower Publishing, 1985).

Robin Gilmour, *The Victorian Period: The Intellectual and Cultural Context of English Literature, 1830–1890* (London: Longmans, 1993).

Pat Jalland, *Death in the Victorian Family* (Oxford: Oxford University Press, 1996).

David B. Morris, *The Culture of Pain* (Berkeley and Los Angeles: University of California Press 1991).

Martin J. Wiener, *Reconstructing the Criminal: Culture, Law and Policy in England, 1830–1914* (Cambridge: Cambridge University Press, 1994).

——, *Men of Blood: Violence, Manliness and Criminal Justice in Victorian England* (Cambridge: Cambridge University Press, 2004).

CHAPTER 8: INTO THE
TWENTIETH CENTURY AND BEYOND

Isabelle Bazanger, *Inventing Pain Medicine: From the Laboratory to the Clinic* (New Brunswick, NJ, and London: Rutgers University Press, 1998).

Jennifer Beinart, *A History of the Nuffield Department of Anaesthetics, Oxford 1937–1987* (Oxford: Oxford University Press, 1987).

Thomas B. Boulton, *The Association of Anaesthetists of Great Britain and Ireland 1932–1992 and the Development of the Specialty of Anaesthesia* (London: Association of Anaesthetists of Great Britain and Ireland, 1999).

Peter Drury, 'Anaesthesia in the 1920s', *British Journal of Anaesthesia* 80 (1998), 96–103.

Christopher Lawrence, 'Experiment and Experience in Anaesthesia: Alfred Goodman Levy and Chloroform Death, 1910–1960', in Christopher Lawrence (ed.), *Medical Theory, Surgical Practice: Studies in the History of Surgery* (London: Wellcome Institute Series in the History of Medicine, 1992).

Jonathan Miller, 'Going Unconscious', in Robert B. Silvers (ed.), *Hidden Histories of Science* (New York: New York Review, 1995).

INDEX

Abbott, Edward 24, 25, 30
Abernethy, John 4
Académie de Médicine 18, 31
Académie des Sciences 27, 31
Acton, William 139
Adelphi Theatre 19
Albert, Prince 84, 85, 86, 87, 88, 93, 94
alcohol:
 used as a stimulant 5, 7, 14, 151
 similarity to ether 56
Alcott, Louisa May
 Sketches of Hospital Practice 118–9
Alfred, Prince 96
Alice, Princess 95
Alma
 battle of 105, 106
America 50, 51
 conflict with Mexico 100–1
 founding of Red Cross 120
American Civil War 113–120
 Medical and Surgical History of the War of the Rebellion 113
 American Journal of Medical Sciences 65
American Medical Association 172
Amsterdam 4
amylene:
 deaths from 92–3
anaesthesia and anaesthetics:
 alternative methods of pain control 67

and antisepsis 119, 165–6
and crime 121–46
and humanitarianism/as symbol of progress/mark of civilization 51, 54, 75–6, 149
and gender 63–5
and race 66
and religion 79–80
and war 97–120
aphrodisiacal effects 142
awareness under 146–7, 177, 191
causes problems in surgery 55
contraindications for 61
dangers of 31–2, 55, 56, 57, 58, 77
degrees of 42
fatalities 169, 170, 171, 172, 190
 in WW1 172–4
 in childbirth 75–86, 187
local 153–4
loss of self control 58–9
mechanism 191–2
methods of administration 49, 87, 168–9
post-anaesthetic vomiting 191
protects female modesty 57
satirised in cartoons 59
selective use 54, 61–2
spinal anaesthesia 183
21c. anaesthesia 190–2
anaesthetists 166–7, 178, 182–3

explosions in operating theatre 183
first London operations under
    ether 30
fistulae 59, 92
in operating theatre 38–9, 57
increase under anaesthesia 60
lithotomy/lithotrity 67
mastectomy 1–4, 22
numbers pre-anaesthesia 4
patients fear of 63
patients refuse 60
range in 18/19th centuries 3
risks and propriety of 4
Organe, Geoffrey 177
Osborne, Revd Sydney 105
Osler, William 152–3
oxygen 9, 11, 18, 181

Paget, James 66, 137
pain:
    and religion 8, 61, 149, 153,
        162–4
    and vivisection 149, 155–8
    as moral danger 149, 155, 158,
        160–1
    as problem 14
    as beneficial 154–5
    as physiological risk 35, 42, 59, 61,
        100
    as stimulant in surgery 5, 40, 61,
        99–100
    as warning of disease 6
    medical understandings of 149–53
    of childbirth 8, 76–80
    of death 8, 14, 151–3
    of dentistry 23–4
    shift in ideas of 40
    understandings change 118,
        149–64, 189
Pall Mall Gazette 131, 143, 145
Palmer, William 136
Papper, E. M. 175
paralysis 177
Paris, 1848 riots 101–2
Park Street medical school 56
Parkinson, Ann 40
Pask, Edgar A. 181, 182
Pasteur Institute 159

patients:
    consent to operations 4
    different responses to pain 62–3
    fear of anaesthesia 49, 54, 146–7,
        192
    fear of pain 60, 63
    power of private patients 68
    response to ether 32–3, 56–7
    tolerate risks of chloroform 51
    travel to London for surgery 68
Pearl Harbour 182
Peel, Sir Robert 62
pentothal (thiopental) 178, 182
Pepys, Samuel 3
Petrequin, M. 50, 51
Petrie, Miss 45
Pharmaceutical Society 33
Pirogoff, Nikolai Ivanovich 101, 112,
    120
pharmaceutical industry 187
photography 98
physiology 15, 16, 43, 142, 157
Pickford, James 55
Pimlico Mystery 131–7
Pinson, K. B. 183
Pneumatic Institute 11, 14
poisons:
    public fear of 125
polio 181, 187
Pope Pius XII 189
Porter, John B. 55, 65, 101, 118
post-mortems 48
Potter, Mary 76
Prescott, Frederick 177
Price, Mr 92
Priestley, Joseph 9, 10, 11, 17, 36
Primatt, Humphry
    A Dissertation on the Duty of Mercy
        and the Sin of Cruelty to Brute
        Animals 16
Pringle, John 9
prostitution 143–4
prussic acid 126
psychiatry 57, 176
public hangings 148, 149, 159–61
Punjab, 2nd Sikh war 102